THE RECOVERY PRESCRIPTION

What Addiction Can Teach Us About Fixing A Broken Healthcare System

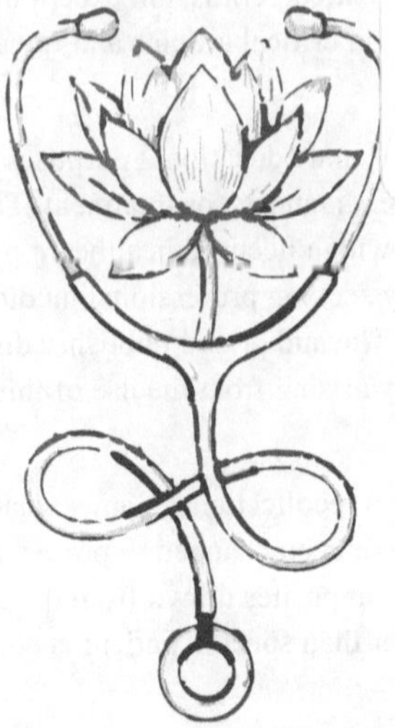

A RECOVERING HEALTHCARE BOOK

THE RECOVERY PRESCRIPTION

Medical Disclaimer
This book is for informational and educational purposes only and does not constitute medical advice, diagnosis, or treatment. The content is not a substitute for consultation with a licensed healthcare provider. Readers should not disregard or delay seeking professional medical advice based on information in this book. The author and publisher disclaim any liability for any loss or injury arising from the use of this information.

Publisher's Note
This work reflects the author's recollections. Names, places, and identifying characteristics have been changed to protect privacy. Many clinical scenarios are composites drawn from the author's professional experience rather than specific patient encounters.

Contact Information
For inquiries, please contact the author at: anthonyjgrandelis@gmail.com

ISBN:
979-8-9937129-4-9 (Hardcover)
979-8-9937129-3-2 (Paperback)
979-8-9937129-5-6 (E-book)

Credits:
Published in the United States by Park Avenue Press
Website: www.parkavenuepress.nyc
E-mail: info@parkavenuepress.nyc

Cover design, typesetting, and e-book formatting by Victor Marcos

First Edition: 2026

To Alex, Alicia, Amy, Jill, Katelyn,
Melinda, Meredith, & Paige

Thank you for helping me feel seen and held
when medical training felt isolating,
and thank you for reminding me, time and again,
that I belong.

I would not have made it through without you,
and your presence has profoundly shaped both
the physician and the person I've become.

Contents

DISCLOSURE

This book reflects the author's present recollections of experiences over time. The events, places, and conversations in this book have been recreated from memory. The chronology of some events has been compressed. When necessary, the names and identifying characteristics of individuals and places have been changed to maintain anonymity and protect their privacy. The majority of clinical scenarios are composite stories from the author's years of experience in healthcare rather than specific patient encounters.

This book is intended for informational and educational purposes only. It is not intended to provide medical advice, diagnosis, or treatment. The information contained herein should not be used as a substitute for consultation with a qualified physician or other licensed healthcare provider. Readers should not disregard or delay seeking professional medical advice based on information contained in this book. The author and publisher disclaim any liability for any loss, injury, or damage allegedly arising from the use or misuse of the information presented. The experiences described in this book reflect the author's personal experiences and opinions.

INTRODUCTION

In 2019, I made one of the hardest decisions of my life: I asked for help. I entered treatment for a substance use disorder that had been quietly, steadily shaping much of my adult life. My struggle with addiction intensified during my medical residency, which is what finally prompted me to enter inpatient rehab. What began as an act of survival and surrender became the beginning of a profound transformation.

My path since then has not been linear or perfect. But it has been honest—and deeply humbling. I've learned that recovery isn't about perfection. It's not about becoming someone new. At its heart, recovery is the radical act of accepting yourself exactly as you are. It's a process grounded in healing rather than fixing—one that asks you to sit with discomfort, give up control, and trust in something larger than yourself.

As an OBGYN hospitalist, I resolved to bring the values I'd learned in recovery into every patient encounter, teaching session, and staff meeting. Values like honesty, humility, faith, surrender, service, and community became lived practices that helped me reconnect with patients, mentor with compassion, and lead with authenticity.

However, as I moved more fully into recovery spaces, I began to notice a growing dissonance between what I was learning there and what I experienced each day in medicine; it was the difference between a culture rooted in vulnerability, accountability, and connection, and a system still organized around perfectionism and control.

In theory, medicine should align beautifully with recovery. Both are about healing. Both are about meeting people where they are. But in reality, the values that define recovery are frequently absent from healthcare. Instead, we work in a system that rewards the myth of invulnerability. It prioritizes getting the "right answer" over being trauma-informed or culturally humble. Too often, the result of buying into that system is burnout, isolation, mistrust, inequity, moral injury, and even suicide. This model of healthcare fails our patients more often than we care to admit. And it also fails us as medical professionals and first responders.

The impulse toward control and inflexibility isn't unique to healthcare; I believe it reflects a broader cultural pattern. We are practicing medicine at a time when divisiveness, fear, and dehumanization are on the rise. It's not surprising that these forces have seeped into healthcare as well, weakening our institutions and leaving them sicker in the process. But this cultural moment has also created an opening for another path forward. It's the same path that has saved countless lives in recovery rooms across the country.

Rooted in the principles of addiction recovery, *The Recovery Prescription* offers a practical framework for improving how care is delivered and experienced in the United States. Drawing on concepts such as honesty, integrity, humility, and community, the book shows how these principles can be applied in everyday clinical settings—from exam rooms to hospital wards. The goal is to shift medicine away from an overemphasis on control and performance, and toward holistic healing, presence, and trust. Written for physicians, nurses, mid-level providers, trainees, administrators, and anyone invested in the future of healthcare, this book invites readers to reimagine not only how we practice medicine, but how we relate to one another and experience ourselves within the medical system.

Recovery is one of the most time-tested and globally validated healing models in existence. Taken together, the principles of recovery form a blueprint for a new paradigm that can restore deeper meaning to our work and greater honesty to our relationships within healthcare. Doing the work outlined in these pages will require us to slow down and listen differently so that we can lead differently—while remembering the values that brought us to medicine in the first place.

When I began writing this book, I went back and re-read an oath I took in medical school. Written by my classmates, the words were idealistic and deeply hopeful: *We arrive at the threshold of our chosen profession pledging to preserve our humility, integrity, and all the values which brought us to the practice of medicine. We will engage in honest self-reflection, striving for excellence but acknowledging our limitations, and caring for ourselves as we care for others...*

Reading this passage now, years later, I see it as something even more profound: a quiet manifesto of recovery. Recovery has changed my life. It continues to change me every day. And by implementing the same values and principles, we can also change the way we practice healthcare in this country. Not through grand reform, but through grounded, daily action that transforms the way we show up, the way we speak, and the way we lead.

This isn't an easy shift. It's a daily practice. A re-orientation that requires deep self-reflection and discomfort. But if we commit to applying these principles, even just for today, I truly believe we'll rediscover an age-old way of practicing medicine. One rooted not in power or control, but in presence and humility. One grounded in honesty rather than fear. One that heals.

Together, we can recover healthcare.

HONESTY

My name is Tony. I'm an addict and an alcoholic. I'm also a fellowship-trained physician, a nationally recognized medical educator, an author, a dog dad, a musician, and a gay man living in New York City. I lead teams. I mentor students. I hold hands in delivery rooms. I make hard decisions.

I introduce myself as all of these different identities because in medicine (and in society), we're far too quick to reduce people to a single identity, diagnosis, or label—especially when it's stigmatized. Over the years, I've had various colleagues and supervisors look at me and see not a physician, but a liability. My advocacy for healthcare workers struggling with substance use has been labeled "unprofessional." I've been whispered about in hallways and asked to keep my story quiet for "the comfort of others." In each instance, it became clear to me that these critics were simply afraid of what they did not understand: addiction.

Addiction among healthcare professionals is far more common than most people realize. *Nearly one in five individuals working in healthcare currently struggle with or have a history of substance use.* As shocking as that figure may be, most experts believe it's significantly underreported.

The true number is likely much greater because the stigma around addiction in medicine runs so deep that many people feel it's safer to suffer alone in silence. Though medical professionals have access to well-structured support systems and programs—most with incredibly high success rates—the persistent culture of fear within healthcare institutions often prevails.

We in medicine are terrified of addiction, particularly as it lives within our ranks. And in our fear, we have missed the vitally important lessons that recovery has to teach us. We've also underestimated its power to heal—not just individuals, but entire institutions.

Over the course of my own recovery, I've come to understand something deeply: *I am not a good doctor despite my addiction. I am a great doctor because of my recovery.*

Recovery principles aren't just tools for personal healing. They offer a powerful blueprint for re-humanizing healthcare. And I believe that if we apply them to how we lead, teach, and care for patients, we will harness the power to restore the soul of medicine.

I didn't arrive at these insights through theory or research alone. I learned them by living them.

My Story

I began my career in medicine as a board-certified, fellowship-trained OB-GYN hospitalist, caring for patients during some of the most urgent and high-stakes moments of their lives, including childbirth. My first job out of training was at a world-renowned institution. I'll admit that the prestige mattered to me; I assumed that excellence in reputation would translate into excellence in leadership and culture. The reality, I soon discovered, was far more complicated.

In my first two years, I worked nonstop to make a name for myself. I became involved in departmental initiatives, earned respect from leadership, colleagues, and trainees, and was honored with a national award for medical student education. For the first time in my career, I felt like I had arrived.

However, I began to recognize a clash between my personal values, which had been shaped by recovery, and the culture of my department. That dissonance began shortly after I arrived, when a newspaper article revealed the complicity of my department's leadership in a sexual misconduct scandal involving hundreds of patients. Several people named in that article were my direct colleagues.

When the article came out, there were no apologies or resignations. No one seemed to honestly acknowledge the pain caused or mistakes made. Instead, leadership quietly moved forward and implemented new protocols to address the issue. When I expressed concern, many colleagues told me to keep my head down and let it go. I had expected an honest reckoning, followed by substantive change. But the colleagues in question remained in leadership roles while continuing to avoid accountability.

Next came a pretty devastating moment for me. I watched as a close friend and mentor, an extraordinary educator, was pushed out for insisting that we needed meaningful reform in our department. He poured his heart and soul into improving the educational experience for medical students. But when his efforts threatened the status quo, he was shut out. His departure sent a clear message: ambition and advocacy were threats, not assets.

After a while, I could no longer ignore the red flags, which included a distressing pattern of silence and lack of support. Initiatives to promote wellness were dismissed without serious consideration. The values of honesty and transparency—along with willingness to take responsibility—were definitely *not* on the agenda.

Despite my misgivings, I continued to press forward in my work. But the faster I rose professionally, the harder I fell in my private life. Beneath the professional accomplishments, I was still living with a substance use disorder. I'd been in recovery for almost four years by that point, and I was so proud of how far I'd come. But I fell into the trap of prioritizing work over my recovery. I said "yes" to every assignment and request that came my way until I finally burned out. And then, when life threw personal challenges my way, I turned to drugs again.

When I relapsed, I did what I had encouraged my patients and trainees to do: I asked for help. I was honest about my struggles, even though the risks were clear. I went to leadership and to the physician health committee, an organization I'd long collaborated with, and told them I needed medical leave. There had been no performance concerns or behavior that warranted discipline. But when the hospital administration found out, I was immediately treated like a liability.

The system didn't ask, *"How can we support you?"* It asked, *"How do we manage you?"* Instead of being met with psychological safety, hospital leadership threatened my medical license. They acknowledged that no safety issues had been raised but still implied that the state medical board would review my performance. *If this is what happens when someone is honest and asks for help, what incentive is there to come forward?* I wondered. The stigma wasn't subtle, and it made an already scary situation feel unbearable. Recovery is hard enough. Doing it under a cloud of shame and professional retaliation is something no physician should have to face.

My experience was in no way unique. It happens every day in institutions all across the country. But having physicians in crisis who are afraid to ask for help remains one of the biggest threats to patient safety, in my opinion. If medical professionals are unable to access basic mental health care due to stigma, we risk having impaired providers who, heaven forbid, make mistakes that could cost innocent people their lives. Lack of honesty about the situation doesn't make it disappear; it simply drives it underground. And I refused to participate in that cycle.

In an effort to reduce stigma and advocate for transparency, I sent an email to the resident physicians explaining that I was taking leave for the disease of addiction. I reminded them that it's okay to ask for help and that support exists. The initial response I received was overwhelmingly positive, but when I returned from treatment, the atmosphere had changed. Leadership avoided me. Friends stopped responding. People unfollowed me on social media. I wasn't met with curiosity or compassion. I was met with silence. I later learned that people were afraid to reach out due to the risk of retaliation from the department's higher-ups.

Eventually, I was summoned to a meeting with senior leadership to review a "return to work" agreement. What I read and heard shocked me. My email to residents had been weaponized. I was accused of utilizing power dynamics to push my views regarding addiction onto trainees. My social media advocacy, intended to support struggling healthcare professionals and raise awareness, was mislabeled as "unprofessional." I was instructed to undergo professionalism remediation as a result.

The response from the hospital leadership team appeared to be punishment for daring to speak openly about addiction and recovery. Notably, I seldom discussed my addiction at work and had never pushed my views on anyone. I simply advocated for a healthier approach to mental health treatment for healthcare professionals.

I believe in seeing the good in people. I have faith that most individuals will choose what's right when given the chance. But my department's leadership repeatedly chose silence over accountability, and comfort over courage.

So, I made one of the hardest decisions of my career: I left. I realized I couldn't stay in a situation that forced me to compromise the values that had been so central to my recovery, even as I continued to care deeply about my colleagues and the patients we served.

It's a choice that no dedicated healthcare professional should have to make.

The Culture of Silence

I begin with this story because it illustrates one of the most entrenched and corrosive dynamics in modern healthcare: the culture of silence.

Silence in medicine isn't just about withholding words. It reflects a deeply embedded belief that speaking the truth - about unpleasant topics such as suffering, uncertainty, mistakes, or injustice - is dangerous. It's the fear that naming what's real will cost us our reputation and possibly our jobs. Silence creates an environment where mental health struggles are seen as moral failings, and where vulnerability is equated with being unfit to lead, teach, or care for patients.

This silence isn't benign. It's a force that upholds hierarchy and suppresses the very humanity we need to practice medicine well. Anyone who's paid even passing attention to the state of healthcare in the United States knows this strategy isn't working. Burnout is endemic. Provider suicide is a crisis. Medical error remains a leading cause of death. Patient dissatisfaction is growing as health disparities widen.

The disconnect between what we experience and what we're allowed to express isn't a coincidence. When a system teaches individuals to deny reality, it becomes internalized. Over time, we learn to override our own truth, normalize the unmanageable, and call it professionalism. Recovery begins by undoing that conditioning.

According to the tenets of Alcoholics Anonymous, the first step on the journey to recovery is simple and revolutionary: "*We admitted we were powerless over drugs and alcohol, that our lives had become unmanageable.*"

This is not a declaration of defeat. It's an act of radical honesty. For many, it's the first time they stop pretending. The first time they name the truth they've been avoiding for years. Honesty is the foundation of recovery, because without it, nothing else can begin.

We cannot heal what we will not name.

I remember the moment I was finally honest with myself about my own addiction. It wasn't after my first relapse, or even my second. It was after my third stay in treatment, when the story I kept telling myself—that I wasn't really an addict, that I just needed to be more disciplined—finally collapsed. I had done what many professionals in high-achieving fields do: I wrapped my identity so tightly around my accomplishments that I convinced myself my suffering couldn't be real. After all, I was a doctor. I was functional. I had patients and colleagues who loved me. I didn't "look like" an addict.

But addiction doesn't care what you look like or what degrees you hold. When I finally told the truth to myself and to others, I felt an enormous wave of relief wash over me. It was like I was finally being allowed to exhale after holding my breath for years.

Since then, I've had to practice that same honesty every single day. I have to remind myself that I live with a chronic, relapsing condition. Every time I go to a recovery support group, I introduce myself as an addict and an alcoholic. I speak my truth out loud. I say it for myself, and I say it for others in the room who are still too ashamed to speak their own truth. Through daily acts of honesty, I remind myself that I am responsible for tending to my recovery, for I've learned that honesty isn't a moment. It's a muscle. And in medicine, it's one that's deeply atrophied.

Medica te ipsum

There's a Latin phrase doctors know from our training:

Medica te ipsum. Physician, heal thyself.

But our current system rarely provides the time and space to tend to our own health because our worth is measured primarily by productivity. Like the addict who insists they're fine, the healthcare system keeps patching holes without addressing the leak.

We are part of a system in denial that launches performative wellness initiatives while punishing providers who admit burnout. It recruits DEI officers while ignoring institutional racism. It holds safety reviews that shame rather than educate. It celebrates resilience while offering no reprieve from the suffering that clinicians bear witness to on a regular basis. And just like addiction, the longer this denial goes on, the worse the damage becomes.

Into Practice

How do we begin to change a culture so deeply entrenched in silence? There's no quick fix. However, it starts with a single step: We begin by noticing, by recognizing the small moments of dishonesty that have quietly woven themselves into our day-to-day work. Once we start paying attention, these moments become almost impossible to ignore.

I see them when a micro-aggression happens, and no one says a word. It's apparent when a trainee lies about a conversation with a patient because they're afraid of looking incompetent, or when a colleague masks exhaustion because asking for help feels too risky. These are situations where we all know something isn't right, but we stay silent anyway. We don't intervene or speak up because we've been taught that silence equals strength and that vulnerability is a liability.

Since entering recovery, honesty has become the cornerstone of my life, including my work in the hospital. Every day on labor and delivery, I practice honesty with myself, my colleagues, and my patients. As a person with a substance use disorder, leading with honesty doesn't come naturally to me. In fact, it can be incredibly hard. But like anything in recovery, the more I practice, the more accessible it becomes.

Some of the simplest ways I practice honesty with patients are by acknowledging uncertainty, being transparent about risks, and naming hard truths. Nearly every day, I meet expectant parents who come to labor and delivery with complicated pregnancies. They all ask the same question: "Is my baby going to be okay?"

The easy answer is "yes." And most of the time, that answer will be true. But it's also incomplete. It leaves no room for nuance, unpredictability, or the reality that complications do happen. So instead, I tell the truth. I say, "I can't be 100% certain that everything will unfold exactly as we hope. But I can promise that we will take excellent care of you and your baby, and if something unexpected happens, we will be there with you every step of the way."

And when complications do happen, I disclose them immediately.

I often think about a difficult delivery that happened during my fellowship—a severe shoulder dystocia, which prevented me from delivering the baby. Ultimately, I resolved the problem by manipulating one of the baby's arms. But in doing so, I fractured the humerus. I felt the pop and knew instantly. After ensuring the patient was stable, I told her exactly what had happened. I explained how challenging the delivery was, and I said, "I'm sorry."

Over the years, I've been repeatedly warned not to say "I'm sorry" for medicolegal reasons. But I will never stop saying it. Even when an intervention is necessary to save a life, harm still matters. For me, apologizing is an act of honesty, and I will not compromise that value. And frankly, that kind of transparency likely does more to prevent litigation than any scripted legal advice ever could.

Another way I practice honesty is by saying, "I don't know."

I am an expert in my field, and there is still so much I don't know. Patients still ask questions that stump me. Instead of guessing or offering false reassurance, I say, "I'm not sure, but I will look into that and get back to you." I do the same with trainees. I believe deeply that mentors must model honesty and that admitting uncertainty is critical when educating the next generation of healthcare providers.

Being honest with colleagues has been harder. For years, I was terrified to admit that I felt overwhelmed, anxious, scared, or burned out. Add to that my fear of confrontation, and honesty with colleagues felt nearly impossible.

Recovery changed that. It taught me to name my feelings and advocate for myself by setting appropriate boundaries. Now, I feel secure enough to say, "I'm overwhelmed and can't take this on right now" or "That case really scared me. I wasn't sure the patient was going to make it." I've learned to recognize when I'm out of my depth and ask for help, to offer direct and constructive feedback, and to challenge toxic norms rather than quietly tolerate them.

As a medical educator and mentor, I lead with honesty as well. I share my real story—not just the polished successes, but the struggles. I talk about nearly quitting medical school because I felt worthless as a medical student, and I reflect on my struggle with anxiety, which often kept me from fully engaging during clinical rotations.

I share how I stepped away from residency to tend to my mental health, and why I eventually left an institution to protect my well-being. If I make a clinical mistake, I acknowledge it and say, "Looking back, I would do this differently." I do this in hopes that my trainees will one day feel empowered to be honest with their patients, their colleagues, and themselves.

And finally, I practice honesty with myself.

Every day, I check in with my motives: *Am I acting from integrity, or am I people-pleasing?* I take stock of my mental state, and I acknowledge burnout when it's present. At the end of each day, I reflect on moments when I may have been dishonest with myself or others.

This is how change begins. Not with sweeping reforms or lofty mission statements, but with honesty that is practiced daily, lived imperfectly, and spoken out loud.

Systemic Change

In recovery, honesty is the prerequisite for healing. But in healthcare, it's too often treated as a liability. A system that truly values honesty must begin by creating psychological and structural safety for clinicians to speak openly about burnout, mental health struggles, substance use, fear, uncertainty, and mistakes without fear of punishment, professional retaliation, or reputational harm.

At a practical level, honesty-guided systems explicitly protect clinicians who disclose the need for support. Policies must clearly separate help-seeking from disciplinary action and make that separation visible and trustworthy. Accessing mental health care, requesting leave, or acknowledging impairment should trigger support pathways rather than credentialing threats or professionalism reviews. When clinicians see colleagues punished for telling the truth, silence becomes the rational choice. An honest system understands that untreated distress is the real risk.

Honesty must also be normalized in clinical knowledge and decision-making. Systems that demand constant certainty incentivize guessing, overconfidence, and false reassurance. By contrast, honest systems explicitly allow (and expect) clinicians to say "I don't know" and to ask for help without stigma. This is reinforced through training, supervision, and evaluation. Leaders and educators must model uncertainty openly, demonstrate how to look things up, and reward curiosity over performance. When uncertainty is named, learning accelerates and patient trust deepens.

Equally important is giving institutional permission to say, "I'm sorry." Despite decades of evidence that transparency and apology improve trust and reduce harm, many healthcare systems still implicitly discourage apology out of fear of legal liability. Honesty-guided systems reject this contradiction. They train clinicians in disclosure and apology as ethical practices, support them when harm occurs, and stand behind them when they speak truthfully to patients and families. Saying "I'm sorry" is not framed as an admission of incompetence, but as an act of integrity and respect. When apology is normalized, accountability becomes relational rather than punitive.

Honesty cannot stop at the bedside; it must extend upward into leadership. Systems guided by honesty require leaders to name institutional harms openly, whether related to misconduct, inequity, unsafe staffing, or toxic culture. Silence, deflection, and quiet policy changes without accountability only deepen mistrust. Honest leadership means apologizing when institutions cause harm and taking responsibility rather than protecting reputations. Without this, calls for transparency ring hollow.

Finally, honesty demands that healthcare institutions tell the truth about the state of healthcare itself. Burnout, moral injury, staffing shortages, and emotional exhaustion cannot be addressed solely through mindfulness apps and resilience workshops. Honest systems name these realities publicly, measure them meaningfully, and commit resources to structural change. It's time to stop pretending that clinicians are broken and instead acknowledge that many are responding normally to unmanageable conditions. This kind of honesty is uncomfortable, but it's also the only starting point for real reform.

In recovery, healing begins when denial ends. The same is true for healthcare. We cannot fix what we refuse to name. Systems guided by honesty don't demand that clinicians carry unbearable truths alone. They create environments where truth can be spoken without fear, where vulnerability is met with support, and where integrity is valued over image. This isn't just a cultural shift. It's a patient safety imperative.

Final Thoughts

Practicing honesty in medicine takes guts. It requires standing in the tension between what is expected and what is real. It demands the willingness to be misunderstood, to be vulnerable, to be seen. And it is also the key to transformation. Because when we're honest with ourselves, our patients, and each other, we can finally make space for healing.

Reflection Questions

1. When was the last time you withheld the truth about your limits, your fears, or your needs because you felt unsafe doing so?
2. What does honesty mean to you in your daily practice? Where are you living in alignment, and where are you not?
3. Have you ever witnessed someone at work who was punished for telling the truth? What message did that send?
4. What conversations are you avoiding right now? What might shift if you approached them with courage and compassion?
5. What stories from your own life, especially those shaped by struggle, might help others feel less alone?

THE PRESENT MOMENT

My Aunt Cindy was only 68 years old when she suffered a stroke. Her health had been deteriorating for years, partly due to alcohol and cigarettes, but also due to a longstanding mistrust of the healthcare system. She'd tried to quit smoking countless times, but nothing ever worked for long. Years of tobacco use and untreated chronic conditions culminated in severe cardiovascular disease and, ultimately, a clot that traveled to her brain.

Cindy didn't often seek medical attention, but when she did, she found herself caught in a system that ultimately validated her fears.

After she had her stroke, she spent seven weeks in and out of three different hospitals. At first, she was sent home (despite her body being half-paralyzed) after doctors somehow concluded she hadn't had a stroke. The second hospital shuffled her between inpatient units and rehab facilities. Her family, overwhelmed and confused, received conflicting information every few days. Every update came from a new physician with a new plan and a new set of medical jargon. There was no continuity of care. No one slowed down to explain the reality of what was happening.

I wasn't living in the state at the time, but I felt the chaos through my mom. I could hear the exhaustion in her voice. Based on what I knew of Cindy's health, I was fairly certain she wouldn't recover, and I suspected she might not live more than a few months. But no one else in our family knew that. And I don't think that's because they were in denial. I think it's because no one on the care team had the time or bandwidth to sit down and tell them the truth.

One day, my mom told me that Cindy was in agony from leg spasms. She would scream out in pain, begging for relief, but she was offered almost nothing. The care team, perhaps influenced by her history of alcohol and tobacco use, refused to treat her symptoms with adequate medication, citing fears of "addiction." Instead of managing her pain or exploring comfort measures, they fixated on hypothetical discharge plans, plans that were never going to happen.

And no one, not once, paused to ask: *Are you scared? Are you in pain? What matters to you right now?*

Four weeks into this, I asked my mom what palliative care had recommended. Her response stopped me cold: *Palliative care hadn't been consulted.* Somehow, in the flurry of consults and chaos, the most essential team, the one that could have brought clarity, comfort, and compassion, was left out.

If you've ever worked with palliative care clinicians, you know their role is sacred. They don't ask what can be fixed.

They ask how they can walk with you, soothe you, and hold space for you, regardless of the outcome. They align care with your goals, not the system's mandates. They are medicine's answer to suffering when a cure is no longer possible. They are stewards of the present moment.

Eventually, Cindy's team did slow down. They finally brought palliative care in after I encouraged my mom to request a consult. Her pain was better managed. Her family finally understood the gravity of her condition. And Cindy, after seven long, frustrating weeks, was finally able to be present with her family. She passed away peacefully in the hospital.

Watching this unfold, even from afar, broke my heart. But as a clinician, it also enraged me. I saw with absolute clarity how difficult it has become for us to truly be with our patients. We're constantly pulled in a dozen directions, answering pages, charting, remembering protocols, and meeting quotas. And somewhere in that chaos, we forget to look up and acknowledge the humanity of the people sitting in front of us. We forget to listen. In our rush, we miss the sacredness of the present moment.

Modern medicine relentlessly focuses on the physical: on fixing, predicting, and preventing. But in doing so, we've neglected something equally vital: the patient's spirit. Human beings are not machines to be repaired. They are souls who experience illness with their bodies, minds, and spirits intertwined. And when we fail to be present, we abandon the part of them that sometimes needs healing the most.

This is a call to return to the bedside and to the human beings in front of us. Because that's where medicine still lives. That's where trust is built and where healing happens, even when curing doesn't. Let's not wait until the end to give our patients the presence they've deserved all along.

Are You Present With Your Patients?

When was the last time you paused before walking into a patient's room, taking a deep breath to ground yourself, instead of rushing through a checklist on autopilot?

When did you last notice the color of your patient's eyes, or the way their voice softened or cracked when speaking of their fears?

When was the last time you sat down while talking with a patient, signaling without words that you weren't in a hurry to leave?

When was the last time you held a patient's hand, not as a clinical gesture, but as a human one?

When was the last time you were fully focused on one patient, without your mind darting to the next task, the next note, the next problem?

When was the last time you noticed your own emotions rise during an encounter? Did you let them pass without judgment? Did you suppress them?

These are hard questions. Ones that ask us to examine our willingness to forge human connections. Each one asks, "Are you prepared to be fully present?"

One Day at a Time

"*One day at a time*" is a common mantra in recovery circles because addicts are experts at time-traveling - replaying past regrets or fantasizing about future escapes. And often, it's this penchant for leaving the present moment that spirals us into relapse. When we leave today, we lose our anchor.

In recovery, when I am consumed by shame about the past, I begin to believe I am irredeemable. When I am fixated on the future, I disconnect from the tools and support available to me right now. The present moment is the only place where recovery actually happens. It is where choice lives. It is where my breath can slow, and my perspective can return. It's where support can be reached. Without the grounding of the present moment, I become untethered and vulnerable to cravings, hopelessness, or impulsivity.

Living in the present moment has always been incredibly difficult for me. I didn't realize why until I was thirty-six years old, when I finally understood that I've lived most of my life with crippling anxiety. For years, I didn't recognize my symptoms as anxiety at all. My internal barometer was my twin sister, who wore her anxiety openly with every outward sign visible as we were growing up. Compared to her, I seemed calm. Functional. Put together. And so I told myself I couldn't possibly be anxious.

WRONG.

What I eventually came to understand was that my constant self-talk—the relentless, looping inner dialogue I assumed was just "thinking"—was actually anxiety. This voice never rested. It was always scanning for danger, judgment, or failure.

Was I smart enough?
Was I attractive enough?
Did people think I was funny?
Would I pass my test?
Would I get into a good college?
Did I play well during my soccer game?
What do my peers really think of me?

It was exhausting. And because it had always been there, I didn't know any other way of being. I wasn't living in the present moment. I was living almost entirely in anticipation, evaluation, and fear.

This unchecked anxiety ultimately followed me straight into medicine. During my years in training, staying present wasn't just difficult. It felt nearly impossible. My mind was constantly racing, caught in an endless loop of worry: *Did my attendings think I was competent? Did I sound intelligent on rounds? Was that piece of feedback a sign I didn't belong?* I lived between rumination over past mistakes and dread of future judgment, rarely anchored in the moment unfolding before me.

These thought patterns were exhausting. Eventually, they progressed beyond being mental noise and became physical burdens. My sleep suffered, my relationships frayed, and my addiction came out of hiding. Even fleeting moments of joy felt dulled by the hum of self-doubt running just beneath the surface. Most painfully, my constant hunger for approval often overshadowed the one thing that mattered most: being fully present with my patients and colleagues.

It wasn't until I got sober that I began to dismantle this cycle.

Recovery taught me what no amount of external praise ever could: that worth is not given to you. It's something you recognize and nurture within yourself.

Slowly, I learned to let go. I began to see that being a good doctor wasn't about accumulating gold stars from supervisors. Rather, it was about showing up fully, honestly, and compassionately for every patient encounter, and being able to look inward and know that I had given my best. I reflected on the small but sacred moments I shared with patients: the tears, the laughter, the silent handholding during devastating conversations. I reminded myself of the hard-earned path that brought me to this place.

I deserved to be here.

Through daily practices like mindfulness and meditation, I learned how to sift through feedback, taking what was useful and letting the rest float away. I learned that my thoughts, no matter how loud or persistent, did not define me. Neither did the passing opinions of others. Staying grounded in the present moment became essential, even when everything around me felt uncertain. And in doing so, I discovered something profound. When I was no longer trapped inside my own fear, I could finally meet my patients (and myself) with the full attention and compassion that true healing demands.

Medicine, for all its technical marvels, had taught me a form of time-travel much like anxiety. As a medical provider, I've been trained to dissect the past for diagnoses and to project the future for prognoses. I've had to plan, to anticipate, to stay two steps ahead. Rarely, if ever, was I taught to simply be with a patient in the present moment. Add in the systemic forces that constantly steal our attention from our patients, and the consequences become quite pronounced.

I cannot tell you how many times I've left a patient's room unable to recall the details of what they said, because my mind was elsewhere - charting in my head, planning my next move, fretting over an outcome I couldn't control. And if my mind was elsewhere, so was my empathy and my care. When we're not fully present, mistakes can happen. Not just clinical errors, but bigger mistakes that fracture trust and steal dignity because they miss the hidden aches patients may not have the words to name.

Narrative Medicine

Narrative medicine offers one of the most profound and necessary shifts in how we approach healthcare today. Developed by Dr. Rita Charon at Columbia University, narrative medicine isn't simply about collecting stories; it is a disciplined practice of deep listening, reflection, and bearing witness to the full complexity of a patient's lived experience. It recognizes that illness isn't just a biological event but a human story, unfolding with emotions, relationships, fears, hopes, and meaning. It's a practice of being present and really hearing our patients.

Narrative medicine teaches healthcare providers to listen beyond symptoms. Patients are invited to share not just what hurts, but who they are and how they are living through their illness. By encouraging patients to elaborate on their lives (their histories, struggles, dreams, and values), providers gain access to critical insights that medical charts and lab results alone could never reveal. These narratives often hold the key to shaping treatment plans that aren't just clinically sound, but also personally meaningful.

But the value of narrative medicine doesn't end with patient care. Engaging deeply with stories invites clinicians into a process of reflection, empathy, and transformation. It reawakens the sense of awe and responsibility that draws most of us to medicine in the first place.

Yet none of this is possible if we, as clinicians, are unable to fully ground ourselves in the present moment. We cannot truly hear a patient's story if we're lost in our own anxieties about what comes next. We cannot honor the vulnerability of another human being if we're distracted or rushed. Presence is the gateway to connection, and connection is the gateway to healing. Thus, narrative medicine calls us back to presence, demanding that we slow down and listen with our whole selves, not just with our ears. Only then can the real work of healing begin.

Into Practice

Staying grounded in the present moment has been one of the hardest recovery principles for me to learn. I am still far from perfect at it, but I've made meaningful progress over the years. The first step was learning to notice when my mind had drifted—into the past, into the future, into worry, judgment, or distraction.

Mindful meditation helped me build that awareness. Even ten minutes a day was enough to see a demonstrable difference in my ability to stay grounded and focused. The core of my practice is simple: noticing my thoughts, acknowledging them without judgment, and gently returning my focus to my breath. Over time, I learned to see thoughts for what they are: impermanent ideas, not commands or truths. The more I practiced letting them go, the easier it became to return to the present moment. That practice slowly began to follow me into my work.

Today, I am very intentional about staying present with patients, and I rely on a few consistent rituals to help anchor me. Before entering a patient's room, I pause at the doorway and take three slow breaths. I set an intention, often something as simple as, "I will let go of what just happened and what comes next, and I will be fully here with this patient."

When I enter the room, I make genuine eye contact and smile before looking at a screen, monitor, or chart. I no longer use a computer during patient encounters, and I have intentionally refused to download the electronic medical record onto my phone. These boundaries protect my attention, and they keep me from disappearing into a screen.

I also make a point to sit down whenever possible. The physical act of sitting slows me down, and it also sends a message: *I'm here. I'm not rushing. You have my attention.* Once that sense of safety is established, I try to learn who my patient is beyond the chart. What's going on at home? What's causing stress right now? What matters most to them today? Who supports them? Is there anyone else who should be part of this conversation?

I also give silence room to breathe. After asking a question, I resist the urge to fill the space. This has been one of the hardest habits for me to change, for silence has always made me uncomfortable. But I've learned that silence tells patients they can take their time. I'm not rushing them toward an answer. And more often than not, the most important truths surface only after a pause.

I also ground myself in sensory details. I feel my feet on the floor. I notice my patient's breathing, their tone of voice, and their posture. When I sense an emotion, I name it aloud: "This feels heavy," or "I can see that you're worried." Naming emotions deepens connection and draws both of us back into the present moment.

Finally, before leaving the room, I summarize what we discussed. I reflect their main concerns, review the plan of care, clarify next steps, and let them know when they can expect follow-up. I ask again if there are any remaining questions. Presence, I've learned, also means clarity.

It doesn't take much for me to do these simple things, but the effect on patient care is astounding. Try some of these practices for yourself, and you'll be amazed at the results.

God Shot

In recovery, a "god shot" refers to an unexpected, deeply meaningful moment. It's a moment that feels like more than a coincidence. One that offers clarity, connection, or reassurance when you didn't know you needed it.

Two years into my first attending job, I walked onto the labor and delivery floor for an overnight shift. As I scanned the board, one name immediately caught my eye: Lacy Mae Moore.

Growing up in the Midwest, one of my closest friends was Michael Moore. We lived on the same cul-de-sac and spent summers running through the neighborhood, letting our imaginations carry us wherever they wanted. Michael had one sister, Lacy Mae.

As we grew older, Michael and I lost touch. Years passed. Then, during my residency, our paths crossed again unexpectedly. I had been caring for a patient with advanced cancer, and one morning during rounds, I recognized a familiar face at the bedside: Mr. Moore. The patient was his sister, Michael's aunt. I remember sitting with them, catching up, laughing briefly in the midst of heartbreak. Michael's aunt passed away shortly thereafter, but that moment stayed with me; it was a quiet reminder that connection could appear where I least expected it.

So, when I saw Lacy Mae Moore on the L&D board years later, my first thought was disbelief. We hadn't seen each other in decades. I had moved to the East Coast, and I didn't even know if she lived in the same city as me. And even if she did, the odds of her being in labor at the exact hospital where I worked, on the exact night of my shift, felt impossible.

Still, I knew something had drawn us together again.

I walked into the room, and there she was. We shared a moment of stunned recognition, followed by a brief, grounding exchange. I asked if she would be comfortable having my colleague manage her labor overnight. I informed her that I'm cautious about caring for friends or family unless absolutely necessary, and she fully supported the plan. I introduced her to the other attending and stepped back.

About an hour later, I glanced up at the fetal heart rate monitoring screen. One tracing stood out immediately: Lacy's. She was experiencing a prolonged fetal bradycardia, which meant that the baby's heart rate had been dangerously slow for an extended period—a warning sign that something was seriously wrong. I asked the resident to check on her, and moments later, an emergency cesarean was called overhead. Her water had broken, and the umbilical cord had prolapsed. It was an obstetric emergency.

In that instant, I understood why our paths had crossed again.

As the team mobilized, I stayed at Lacy's side while we rushed to the operating room. Her family had stepped out briefly, not expecting anything urgent so early in labor. She was alone and scared.

My colleagues were preparing. The other attending was scrubbing in for the surgery. My role was simple: I needed to sit with her, stay present, and remind her she was not alone—that we were doing everything possible to keep her and her baby safe.

Minutes later, her baby boy was born, crying loudly. He was safe, and the rest of the surgery was performed without complications. Later, I met Lacy in the post-surgical recovery unit and had the privilege of calling her parents to tell them their daughter and grandson were both healthy.

That night, I didn't perform the surgery. I didn't make a medical decision that changed the outcome. All I did was stay present. I was a familiar face in a moment of fear and uncertainty. It remains one of the most human moments I've ever shared with a patient, and I am so grateful I was able to be there.

Systemic Change

If we're serious about restoring the present moment to medicine, systemic change requires an honest reckoning with how thoroughly our systems fragment attention. Presence can't survive in environments designed for constant interruption. We cannot ask clinicians to be grounded, attentive, and emotionally available while simultaneously subjecting them to relentless paging, excessive documentation, the constant pull of new technology, rotating teams, and productivity metrics that reward speed over understanding. A system committed to presence would begin by acknowledging that distraction is a predictable outcome of how we have structured modern healthcare. And with that distraction comes worse patient care, both at the clinical and human levels.

One of the most necessary shifts would be redefining time itself as a clinical resource rather than a logistical obstacle. This means building schedules and staffing models that allow clinicians to remain with patients during moments that matter without the constant pressure to move on to the next task. This might even require a complete reimagining of how hospitals bill for care and compensate their providers in the United States.

To bring the providers back to the bedside, and I mean truly present at the bedside, productivity-based models need a dramatic restructuring or need to disappear altogether. A change like this would be challenging in our political system, but perhaps we can learn a little from non-productivity-based systems being utilized in various European countries. Being present with a patient is an intervention that is as important as any other drug, procedure, or test.

Documentation must also be redesigned to serve care, not eclipse it. Electronic medical records should function as tools for continuity and clarity, rather than creating constant demands on attention during human encounters. Systems that value presence would encourage clinicians to look up, sit down, and listen. This might mean reducing redundant documentation, separating billing from clinical notes, or creating team-based documentation models that allow one person to chart while another remains at the bedside. This also might look like removing computers from the exam room altogether. Believe it or not, this is how medicine was practiced for years.

Another important way to protect presence is to rethink how we communicate with one another in the hospital. Most institutions now rely on secure text messaging platforms or dedicated work phones, both of which demand immediate attention and pull clinicians out of the room, sometimes literally and always cognitively. The moment a text appears on screen, our focus shifts. We read the message, start mentally triaging a new task, and disengage from the patient in front of us, even when the issue is not urgent. Phone calls are no better; they require immediate interruption by design. The vast majority of these communications are not emergencies and could safely wait, yet our systems are built around instant response, reinforcing a culture of constant urgency that exhausts everyone.

We've grown so accustomed to immediacy that waiting even a few minutes feels intolerable, and that impatience comes at the cost of connection. What if we reclaimed a slower, more intentional approach? Returning to pagers, for example, would allow clinicians to signal one another without hijacking the present moment, paging a number to return a call or text within a set window unless the situation is truly emergent. Emergencies would still warrant immediate escalation through clearly defined channels. But non-urgent requests would no longer rush us out of meaningful encounters. No clinician should feel pressured to end a patient conversation because of interruptions that can wait. Presence at the bedside should be protected, not constantly negotiated away.

Continuity of care must also be reclaimed. When patients are passed from one provider to another, day after day, the burden of storytelling falls on those who are already exhausted and frightened. Systems built for presence would prioritize stable, team-based models that know the patient beyond their problem list and can hold the arc of their story. Fewer handoffs, clearer communication across teams, and deliberate transitions of care are acts of respect for the patient's lived experience.

Early and automatic integration of palliative care is another essential structural change. Palliative care shouldn't be viewed as a consult of last resort, triggered only when death feels imminent. Instead, systems should embed palliative principles (symptom management, goal alignment, emotional support) into routine care for patients with serious illness. They should be a part of EVERY checklist or protocol. Automatic triggers based on clinical criteria, repeated hospitalizations, uncontrolled pain, or caregiver distress would ensure that presence enters the room before suffering becomes normalized. This would prevent scenarios like my aunt Cindy's, where weeks pass before anyone pauses to ask what matters now.

Final Thoughts

Reclaiming the present moment in medicine isn't about slowing everything down indiscriminately. It's about slowing down where it matters most. It's about recognizing that healing doesn't only happen through interventions aimed at the future, but through attention offered now. When systems are designed to protect presence, we make room for a different kind of medicine to emerge. One that reminds us that the work we do is not only about saving lives – it's about being fully human in the moments that matter most.

Reflection Questions

1. When was the last time you were fully present with a patient? What did that feel like in your body and your mind?
2. What tends to pull you away from the present moment during clinical encounters? During conversations with colleagues?
3. How often do you pause and breathe before moving from one task or room to the next? What changes when you do?
4. Do you allow space for silence and emotional reflection in your conversations with patients, trainees, and/or colleagues?
5. Outside of work, how do you cultivate mindfulness?

SURRENDER

I was born and raised in the Midwest and completed all of my medical training there: medical school, residency, and fellowship. When I graduated and accepted a position at an academic institution on the East Coast, I knew I was stepping into a new chapter. I'd been warned, more than once, about how different the culture of obstetrics would be in the Northeast. I thought I was prepared. I was wrong.

The shift was more than geographic. It was existential.

As a fellowship-trained OBGYN hospitalist, I have a deep passion for quality improvement and patient safety. I've always believed that we can make birth safer, more equitable, and more humane through reflection, process evaluation, and systemic change. With the rising rates of maternal mortality in the United States, I've always seen quality work as an essential part of my responsibilities. But when I started my first attending job, I quickly realized that the quality and safety culture wasn't focused on improvement. It was obsessed with control.

There's an important difference between improving outcomes and controlling them.

Improvement asks: *How can we make things safer for patients and more sustainable for providers?*

Control demands: *How can we prevent every single bad thing from ever happening, no matter the cost?*

And that cost, as I would learn, is high.

Each month, our institution held safety review meetings to discuss adverse outcomes. These meetings were massive. Dozens of providers in a room, analyzing case after case. What stunned me most wasn't just the volume of reviews, but the format. In every case, we were essentially asked to vote on whether the provider involved was "at fault" and whether that fault was inherent to that provider's clinical capabilities.

The provider's identity was supposed to be anonymous, but it rarely was. Gossip moved faster than any safety committee memo. And the accused provider wasn't even allowed to be present. They had no opportunity to explain their reasoning or the context of the moment to their peers. It felt less like a professional learning environment and more like a tribunal.

Unsurprisingly, the consequences rippled far beyond that room. Fear saturated the air. Practitioners practiced defensively, not because it was evidence-based, but because it was safe for them. Every questionable fetal heart rate strip, every deviation from protocol became grounds for panic. It seemed as though cesarean deliveries were being performed for provider protection, not fetal benefit.

We weren't improving care. We were drowning in a sea of anxiety, bureaucracy, and self-protection. The very culture that was supposed to safeguard patients was, instead, eroding provider well-being and worsening the patient experience.

One glaring example of this obsession with control came in the form of a very expensive artificial intelligence software that our hospital purchased to monitor fetal heart rate tracings. If you're not familiar, continuous fetal monitoring is one of the most commonly used tools in labor and delivery units across the United States. It is meant to assess fetal wellbeing in real time, but there's little evidence that it improves outcomes, particularly in uncomplicated pregnancies. In fact, it may do the opposite by increasing our cesarean delivery rates due to over-interpretation and misinterpretation of "non-reassuring" patterns, which don't necessarily predict poor outcomes. Yet instead of reckoning with this complexity, our institution doubled down by throwing money at a high-tech solution to give us the illusion of more precise control.

The problem wasn't that we were using technology. The problem, in my opinion, was that we were using it to medicate our fear rather than improve care. We were chasing control in the rarest, most unpredictable cases, while causing more harm in the common, preventable ones. I became increasingly worried that we were heading towards more unnecessary cesareans, increased maternal and neonatal morbidity, more provider burnout, and more patients feeling unheard and over-medicalized.

All the while, we told ourselves it was about "safety." But what we were really doing was reacting to our fear of bad outcomes, lawsuits, public blame, and reputational harm. We were mistaking control for care. That confusion runs deep, not just in obstetrics, but across all of healthcare.

Control and Recovery

One of the foundational lessons I've learned in recovery is that control is an illusion. As someone with a substance use disorder, I tried to control everything. I tried to control my emotions with substances. I tried to control others' perception of me. I tried to control my use (just a little, just this once, just one more time) even when the consequences were devastating. I tried to control the outcome of almost any interaction in my life, getting angry whenever things didn't go my way. And the harder I tried to control my environment, the more anxious, paranoid, and disconnected I became. It took me a long time to learn that I am not actually in control of most things in my life, and that trying to control the uncontrollable is a recipe for suffering.

In *The Untethered Soul*, author Michael Singer writes about how ridiculous it is, in the grand scheme of the cosmos, to believe we can control anything. We're one of billions of humans, on a planet spinning through a vast universe, and yet we always convince ourselves that if we just try hard enough, we can make everything go our way. This belief isn't just false. It's dangerous. It leads to overreaction, rigidity, and despair when things don't go exactly as we plan.

In recovery, I've discovered a different way. I practice acceptance and surrender, learning to respond instead of react. I've stopped trying to force outcomes, and I now show up with intention, presence, and humility. I repeat the Serenity Prayer daily for a reason:

Grant me the serenity to accept the things I cannot change,
The courage to change the things I can,
And the wisdom to know the difference.

Giving Up Control in Medicine

The longer I've been in recovery, the more I've become acutely aware of how desperately we cling to control in medicine. Every day, I watch my colleagues, trainees, and other staff members trying to control things that they cannot. Ultimately, they become frustrated and overwhelmed when things don't go as they planned.

One of the most common examples is when patients don't take our medical advice. During my training, I began to realize that what appears to be noncompliance often has a story behind it—one that rarely fits neatly into our clinical frameworks. This was the case for a patient of mine named Amina.

Amina was a 32-year-old Somali woman, a mother of five who was pregnant with her sixth. She'd been referred to our hospital for urgent inpatient management of uncontrolled diabetes in pregnancy. Amina was soft-spoken and calm in a way that unsettled us, given the gravity of her condition. Her blood sugars were dangerously high, her amniotic fluid levels were elevated, and the fetus was measuring weeks ahead—details that carried an ominous weight for any obstetrician. We feared stillbirth. We feared shoulder dystocia. We feared preeclampsia, diabetic ketoacidosis, ICU admissions, and devastating loss.

Amina, however, was not afraid.

She sat upright on the exam table, her hands folded in her lap. When we explained the risks to her for the third time, she nodded, her expression unchanged.

"I understand," she said. "But I will not stay in the hospital."

I leaned forward. "Amina, I know this isn't what you were expecting today. But the risk to you and your baby is very real. We're trying to help. You could get very sick. So could the baby."

"I understand," she said again, her voice steady. "But I need to be home. My children need me. My husband is at work. There is no one else. I trust in Allah. If this baby is meant to live, the baby will live."

There was no anger in her voice. No defiance. Just a quiet certainty that disarmed us.

The team froze. The nurses exchanged glances. Someone tried again to explain what she was risking. We emphasized that it wasn't just her life, it was her baby's, too. That if she came back in crisis, it might be too late.

She listened carefully. Then she smiled. A kind, tired smile. And she said, "Everything is already written."

We weren't uncomfortable because we didn't understand her values, but because we could not control the outcome. We were trained to manage complications, not to surrender to them. Our role was to act, intervene, prevent, save. And when a patient like Amina looked us in the eye and said, "I do not want saving," it broke the spell we were taught to live under: the illusion that we are in control.

She had capacity. She was clear about her situation and had understood everything we told her. And she still said no.

In the hallway, someone muttered, "What kind of mother risks her baby like that?" But I found myself thinking: *What kind of system refuses to believe that faith and family are valid reasons to go home?*

Amina did not need saving. She needed to be seen. And she needed us to respect that this was her life—her body, her child, her decision. Not ours.

Amina reminded me of something I had forgotten in the rush of protocols and fear: all of life is temporary. All of it. We are not here to prevent death. We are here to honor life, however our patients define it. Sometimes, that means doing everything we can. And sometimes, that means letting go of what we think is best. Sometimes it means bearing witness rather than intervening. And sometimes, it means saying goodbye to someone who walks out of our hospital and into the hands of their God, trusting that they are choosing a kind of safety we cannot offer.

The story above illustrates one of the most difficult truths in medicine: we cannot control patient decisions. No matter how well we explain or how passionately we recommend a course of action, the decision ultimately belongs to the patient, not to us.

And yet, we try. Desperately.

Take patient follow-up, for example. In OBGYN, we often manage patients with a pregnancy of unknown location (when the pregnancy is too early to be visualized on ultrasound). We follow the beta-hCG hormone serially, trying to determine whether the pregnancy is viable or ectopic.

We carefully explain everything to the patient. We counsel them about signs of ectopic rupture: dizziness, pain, and fainting. We tell them to return in 48 hours, add them to follow-up lists, and set reminders. If they don't return, we call. And call. And call again. We leave voicemail after voicemail. If they answer, we repeat the same script, trying to pin them down for a return time. We double down on documentation and compliance workflows.

All the while, we are chasing an outcome we do not—and cannot—control.

Patients are autonomous human beings. And when they don't make the choices we want, we try even harder to force them into compliance. The result? More emotional labor. More burnout. More frustration. All without any clear evidence that we're actually improving outcomes.

This obsession with control shows up everywhere. We get frustrated when patients don't disclose their full history, yet fail to acknowledge that they may not feel safe doing so. We label them "poor historians" instead of considering our own failures in communication or trust-building.

We expect immediate behavior change (smoking cessation, dietary adjustments, substance use treatment), but we overlook how complex and nonlinear those changes are. We call patients "non-compliant" rather than recognizing they may be pre-contemplative, ambivalent, or afraid. We roll our eyes when patients reference things they've read on the internet, and we dismiss the advice they've received from loved ones. In doing so, we ignore the entire ecosystem they're navigating outside our exam room.

Even when we follow the playbook perfectly, outcomes can still go wrong.

I will never forget the aftermath of a maternal death at one of the hospitals where I trained. The patient had every possible risk factor for cardiopulmonary complications, including morbid obesity, diabetes, hypertension, asthma, sleep apnea, and preeclampsia. She had a cesarean delivery, decompensated postoperatively, and died in the ICU after a cardiac arrest.

After her death, chaos ensued. The case was labeled "preventable." But was it? No one could say for sure. But labeling it "preventable" gave us something we could cling to. It made us feel like we still had control. If it were preventable, we could fix it.

And so the system reacted. An investigation was launched. Providers were pulled aside and quizzed on protocols. As fear spread, meetings multiplied, and our inboxes were flooded with emails. More compliance training. More reviews. More policies. More control.

But control is an illusion. Bad outcomes sometimes happen. And when they do, our systems react by tightening their grip.

This tendency doesn't stop at patient care. We try to control our colleagues, too, by managing how we're seen and received. But no matter how carefully we calibrate our actions, we can't control how other people respond. Some people will misunderstand us. Some will project their own pain onto our actions. Some will be unkind, no matter how kind we are.

Of course, we cannot control the systems we work in or external circumstances. We can't influence insurance denials, limited budgets, staffing shortages, unavailable medications, or missing equipment. We have limited power over state laws that ban evidence-based care or politicians who legislate medical decisions with no regard for clinical nuance. We have no say over patient volume or acuity.

Whether we like it or not, emergencies, interruptions, and challenges will arise. There's so much in life that we won't be able to fix, despite our best intentions. But we can recognize what is and isn't ours to carry. We can choose to let go of what we cannot control and instead anchor ourselves in what we can.

Into Practice

In recovery, my first act of surrender was admitting to myself that I was powerless over drugs and alcohol. That I couldn't control my use and that I needed help. Since that moment, I've slowly learned to accept things that are out of my control and to re-focus my energy where it can actually make a difference.

In medicine, this shift has been profound. My new mindset has brought a deep sense of peace and purpose to my clinical practice. It's improved my relationships with my colleagues and patients alike and allowed me to be more present in my teaching.

Let me share with you how this principle plays out in my day-to-day work:

I begin each day by controlling how I arrive. I ground myself before walking into the hospital, usually by listening to a meditation on my way into work. During my commute, I set an intention for my day. While I cannot control how busy the unit will be or what emergencies lie ahead, I *can* choose to be present. Before each patient interaction, I center myself by taking a moment to slow down. Then I sit down, make eye contact, and listen without interruption.

I also control how I communicate, choosing clear, compassionate language when explaining complex medical issues. Even under pressure, I soften my tone. I practice inclusive language and ask open-ended questions, creating space for patients to share their whole story. When faced with uncertainty, I allow myself to say, "I don't know." My goal is to remain connected in conversation during times of uncertainty, letting go of the need to have all the answers, all the time. This is a powerful act of surrender that shifts my focus from control to connection.

One of the hardest but most important lessons I've learned is that I'm responsible for my own boundaries. While I cannot control the culture of overwork in medicine, I *can* say "no" when I'm burned out. I *can* advocate for myself and ask for help. I *can* choose rest. I *can* nourish my body. I *can* prioritize joy, hobbies, and relationships outside of medicine. And I *can* treat myself with the same compassion I offer to others.

Another thing I can control is how I respond to feedback. I used to react very defensively to feedback, but recovery has taught me otherwise. Now, I choose to receive honest feedback with curiosity and self-compassion instead of shame. Making this shift has helped me to reflect and grow.

I also control how I handle conflict. Disagreements in medicine are inevitable. What I *can* control is my response. I no longer rush to judgment or immediately escalate. Rather, I practice empathy. I lead with open-mindedness and try to understand before being understood. I ask myself what matters more: being "right" or maintaining a positive working relationship with the person I am in disagreement with?

It's up to me to choose how I lead and how I show up for my team. Every colleague, regardless of title, deserves to be treated with dignity and respect. I advocate for those without a voice and support junior team members. Even when I'm tired, I lead with empathy. My focus is on building people up, not wearing them down. And when systems fail our patients, I fight for change.

SYSTEMIC CHANGE

Systemic change, in the context of surrender, would look like healthcare finally admitting what every seasoned clinician already knows in their bones: uncertainty is not a defect in the system. It is the natural condition of medicine. We cannot design institutions around the fantasy of total control without traumatizing the people who work inside them and harming the people they serve. A surrender-informed system would still be relentless about safety, but it would replace fear-driven vigilance with humility-driven learning. It would stop treating adverse outcomes as failures of the individual and instead treat them as opportunities to recognize patterns in complications.

It's also crucially important to build a "just culture" that distinguishes human error from reckless behavior and invites the involved clinicians into the review process rather than banishing them from it. Our peer reviews would be structured around questions like, "What did the system make hard?" and "Where did our processes fail the clinician and the patient?" Questions about the provider would be removed entirely, unless reckless behavior was clearly identified.

A system practicing surrender would also interrogate its own addiction to metrics, surveillance, and technological fixes that soothe institutional anxiety without improving outcomes. It would ask hard questions such as: *Are we using our tools (like fetal monitoring algorithms) to micromanage uncertainty while ignoring the downstream harms of over-intervention, loss of patient autonomy, and defensive practice patterns?*

Making these shifts would create team-based decision-making structures that distribute responsibility so that no single clinician feels forced to make a decision to protect themselves. In other words, it would stop rewarding control and start rewarding calibration, nuanced risk assessment, honest communication, and restraint when restraint is the safest choice.

Systemic surrender would also fundamentally reshape how healthcare relates to patients, moving us toward effective partnership. In recovery, surrender doesn't mean giving up responsibility; it means releasing the illusion that we can—or should—coerce outcomes. Applied to healthcare systems, this requires abandoning policies built around patient compliance and replacing them with structures that honor patient autonomy as an ethical anchor rather than a liability. When care is organized around obedience, refusal becomes a threat to be managed. But when care is organized around partnership, refusal becomes information—an expression of values, fears, and priorities that deserves respect and curiosity.

One of the clearest places this shift could occur is in how we handle decisions traditionally labeled as "against medical advice." The term itself carries moral judgment and institutional defensiveness, framing patients as defiant rather than discerning. A system grounded in surrender would eliminate this language, along with the punitive paperwork that often accompanies it. Instead, these encounters would be documented simply and honestly: that risks, benefits, and alternatives were discussed, that the patient demonstrated understanding, and that an autonomous decision was made. No extra forms. No escalation. No implicit threat. This reframing acknowledges a fundamental truth: informed adults are allowed to make choices that clinicians would not choose for them.

A hospital that practices surrender understands that the goal is not to eliminate all bad outcomes; it is to create a system that responds to outcomes with learning rather than blame, presence rather than panic, and compassion rather than control. That is what it looks like when medicine stops trying to be omnipotent and starts becoming wise.

Final Thoughts

Control is deeply woven into the fabric of modern medicine.

We are trained to predict, prevent, and protect. To be vigilant and infallible. We measure success by the ability to fix. And yet, the deeper we go into this work, the more we come to see that so much of it lies beyond our reach.

Sometimes patients make decisions we wouldn't make. And sometimes outcomes defy logic. Bodies don't behave like textbooks. Systems fail. Grief comes. And control slips through our fingers again and again.

Practicing surrender in medicine doesn't mean we stop striving for excellence. It means we stop confusing control with care. It means we recognize that our patients' bodies, beliefs, and decisions are not ours to manage. We cannot mold them to fit our preferences. We must meet people where they are, not where we want them to be.

In the end, surrender is about showing up with less fear and more humility. It requires us to cultivate a deeper respect for the mystery of life and death. Because the truth is that all of this is temporary, and we do not save anyone. We walk beside them. We do our best. And then we must let go.

Reflection Questions

1. Where in your practice do you notice a need for control over outcomes, patients, or colleagues?
2. How does your fear of bad outcomes impact your decision-making?
3. Can you recall a time when surrender (accepting what you could not change) led to more clarity, connection, or peace?
4. How might surrender change the way you handle emotionally or ethically complex cases?
5. What is one thing you're holding too tightly right now in your professional life? What might it look like to let go, even slightly?

SAFETY

Angela came into triage at 2:00 a.m. on a Saturday, 30 weeks pregnant and contracting regularly. She was twenty-eight years old. Her chart read: "anxiety, opioid use disorder in remission." Apparently, she was a "frequent flyer," a phrase that says everything about how we'd already decided to see her before she'd said a word. The nurse glanced at me and sighed, "Here we go again…"

It was my first time meeting Angela. I sat beside her and tried to gather a history, but she avoided eye contact and answered in clipped, guarded phrases. When I explained the need for a pelvic exam, given her preterm contractions, she refused. I tried again, gently outlining the clinical risks. Angela still refused. This was her fifth pregnancy. She'd likely had countless pelvic exams. I was perplexed.

I sat down beside her at the bedside, softened my voice, and asked, "Can you tell me what worries you about the exam? Is there anything I can do to make you feel more comfortable?"

She stared at the ceiling. "I just don't want to be examined unless absolutely necessary," she said quietly.

So I didn't. Instead, I obtained her consent to perform an abdominal ultrasound, which showed a minimally dilated cervix and adequate amniotic fluid. We hydrated her with IV fluids, and her contractions slowed. She agreed to self-collect infectious swabs. I kept her admitted for monitoring.

The next day, before she went home, Angela thanked me. "Thank you for not pushing the exam," she said. I told her, "Of course. You never have to do anything you don't feel safe doing."

That's when the story changed.

Angela told me she had been sexually assaulted as a teenager and that she had used opioids to escape the trauma. Her last pregnancy had been marked by withdrawal, judgment, and an emergency cesarean she barely remembered. "I've often felt like my body isn't mine," she said. "Coming here, it feels like I'm just an object. Another chart, another number. And no offense, doctor, but I struggle with male providers."

I told her I understood. I let her know she could request a female provider anytime, and I asked if I could add a note to her chart so her history didn't have to be re-explained every time. She agreed. When she returned two months later in labor, she was met with kindness, boundaries, and care. She delivered a healthy, full-term baby and expressed immense gratitude for the way our team honored her experience.

I think about Angela often. I relate to her story, not only because of my own experience with substance use disorder, but because I know what it feels like to live in a body that doesn't always feel safe or like my own.

Addiction is so often misunderstood. On a biological level, yes, it's a brain disorder involving dysregulated dopamine pathways and hijacked reward systems. And yes, there's often a strong genetic predisposition. But these explanations, while important, don't capture the full truth. Because addiction isn't just about craving, it's about coping. It's about pain.

In recovery communities, you'll often hear people say that nearly everyone carries trauma. Sometimes it's loud (assault, violence, abandonment). Other times, it's quiet (neglect, shame, isolation). But nearly always, addiction begins as a survival mechanism, a way of coping with things that feel unbearable.

The data backs this up. Trauma rewires the brain. It distorts attachment and reshapes the individual's understanding of their self-worth. In fact, over two-thirds of people with substance use disorders report histories of physical or sexual abuse. Additionally, the Adverse Childhood Experiences (ACE) study shows a clear correlation: the more trauma a person experiences in childhood, the higher their risk for addiction, mental illness, and chronic disease.

As Dr. Gabor Maté famously asks, "The question is not why the addiction, but why the pain?"

Trauma in Healthcare

As medical professionals, we experience trauma nearly every day at work. Death, suffering, and injustice surround us, often with little space to process what we've witnessed. At times, we are blamed—or even sued—for doing our best under impossible conditions. We're punished for showing emotion and praised for stoicism, which trains us to override our own physical, emotional, and spiritual needs in the name of professionalism.

It's trauma by attrition. One thousand paper cuts to the soul, leading to a quiet erosion of emotional and moral resilience. And we cope in many of the same ways that our patients do, through disengagement, overworking, emotional detachment, and even substances. We say, "I'm fine," when we're not, and we brush aside our own feelings with the rationalization, *"Well, this is what I signed up for."* Ultimately, we become providers who see trauma in others, but not in ourselves.

It's tempting to think of psychological safety and trauma-informed care as something we do for patients, like adopting a new script, following a checklist, or completing a training module. But in reality, it's a way of being. And it starts with our own stories. It starts with asking: *What happened to me? How do I respond when I feel powerless? What's underneath my own anger, numbness, defensiveness, or need to fix?*

We cannot offer safety to others until we create it within ourselves. When we do our own work, through therapy, reflection, recovery, or peer support, a change occurs. We learn to tolerate uncertainty without grasping for control. We begin to soften our judgments of ourselves, our patients, and our colleagues. We start to show up with curiosity instead of shame.

Of course, individual reflection isn't enough. We must also continue to advocate for a culture of medicine that acknowledges trauma among providers, as well as the fact that our systems often perpetuate it. That means pushing back on shaming feedback styles, toxic perfectionism, and unattainable standards. We must refuse to remain silent about suicide, depression, or addiction among providers and hierarchies that discourage vulnerability. It means asking, *"Are we designing systems that mirror healing or systems that mirror trauma?"*

In recovery, we say, "You're only as sick as your secrets." Medicine has many secrets. Clinicians don't talk about the trauma we experience at work. We don't talk about shame. We don't talk about imposter syndrome or the emotional toll of practicing medicine. But we can start.

Into Practice

For me, learning to practice trauma-informed care and create psychological safety for my patients didn't begin with a course or a framework. It began in recovery, when I was finally forced to look inward.

Early in my recovery, I was asked to examine my own history honestly: not just what had happened to me, but how I had learned to survive. I began to see how my identity, upbringing, and lived experiences shaped the way I responded to stress, criticism, and conflict, both in medicine and in life.

In my own experience, the trauma was quiet. Subtle. It lived in the silence of things not said. Before I ever picked up a drink or used a drug, I learned what it meant to feel wrong in my own skin.

Growing up in the Midwest, I was a creative kid who loved theater, music, and art. I loved being around girls, but not in the way boys were "supposed" to. From early on, I sensed I was different. And while my family wasn't overtly homophobic, there was a glaring absence of any positive LGBTQ+ messaging. Mind you, I grew up in the 90s when "gay" was a common slur used amongst children and adolescents.

I was so afraid of being gay—of being different—that I tried to hide it at all costs. I became a master of achievement, using success to stay invisible: a straight-A student, varsity athlete, student leader, musician, and pre-med. If I could do enough, maybe no one would notice how much I hated myself. Maybe I wouldn't notice either. On the outside, it looked like I was doing just fine. But inside, I was carrying a wound I didn't have words for - the trauma of erasure.

The trauma wasn't physical, and there wasn't one defining event that explained it all. It was the slow, corrosive message that who I was at my core wasn't okay and that love was conditional. The message I received was that I had to hide my true identity to stay safe. For years, I believed that if I could control how others saw me, I might finally belong. This survival strategy followed me into adulthood and ultimately into medicine.

Because of it, I developed a deeply unhealthy relationship with feedback. Any criticism, no matter how small, felt like a judgment of my worth. I didn't hear information; I heard rejection. Shame flooded in quickly. Sometimes I lashed out defensively. Other times, I withdrew completely, replaying the interaction in my head for days, convinced I wasn't good enough.

Medical training only reinforced these patterns. I remember vividly being a resident learning a minimally invasive hysterectomy with a notoriously harsh attending. As I struggled with part of the procedure, she announced to the entire operating room that her two-year-old had better spatial awareness than I did. I felt exposed and humiliated. I carried that comment with me for years, internalizing it as proof that I didn't measure up.

Over time, fear of criticism made learning harder. I avoided opportunities where I might fail. As a direct result, I became emotionally numb and increasingly detached over time. Eventually, substances became a way to quiet the shame and anxiety I didn't yet have language for.

My experience of trauma didn't end there. Substance use, in and of itself, is a terrible form of physical, mental, and emotional trauma that addicts inflict upon themselves. And I also experienced relationship trauma in the form of physical and emotional abuse.

Despite all this, I was able to convince myself for a very long time that I hadn't experienced any trauma at all. However, recovery taught me something medicine never had. It helped me understand that trauma has infinite forms. For me, trauma lived in chronic shame and in repeated experiences of humiliation in environments where safety felt conditional.

Once I understood that, I began to see my patients differently. They were no longer problems to solve, but people shaped by experiences I could not see. I realized that every patient carries trauma to some degree, and that, sometimes, trauma can profoundly shape how they experience healthcare.

Recovery also taught me a humbling truth: it is not my job to diagnose or fix trauma. My role is simpler and more important. My job is to create conditions of psychological safety, dignity, and empowerment so patients can fully engage in their own care. That understanding shows up in small, intentional ways every day.

I greet patients with warmth and presence. I make eye contact, and I introduce myself clearly. I explain what will happen before it happens. During exams or procedures, I describe each step in advance and remind patients that we can stop at any time. I repeatedly ask for consent—not just once—saying, "Are you still okay to continue?"

I offer options whenever possible. For example, I routinely tell my patients, "There are a few ways we can approach this. Let me walk you through them." I name power dynamics out loud, "This is a partnership, and your voice matters here."

When patients become tearful or withdrawn, I don't rush to fix or redirect. I validate their experience by saying, "It makes sense that this feels overwhelming. I'm here with you." I resist labeling patients as "difficult" or "non-compliant," and instead get curious about what might be happening beneath the surface. I use respectful, non-stigmatizing language, and I model that same compassion in handoffs and team discussions.

And I intentionally lift patients up by telling them, "You've done a lot to get here today," or "It's clear how much you care about your health and your family." I ask about their support systems and about barriers that might make seeking care more difficult (transportation, food, safety) because trauma-informed care doesn't stop at the exam table.

Creating psychological safety for trainees is also of paramount importance. I do this by making it unmistakably clear that learning matters more than perfection. I model humility by naming my own uncertainty, normalizing question-asking, and reframing mistakes as learning opportunities. Trainees know they can speak up around me because I listen without interruption and give feedback that is grounded in respect. I pay attention to power dynamics and intentionally flatten hierarchies so everyone feels equally empowered to raise concerns in the moments that matter most. By consistently protecting learners from ridicule, advocating for them when systems fail, and holding high expectations within a framework of trust, I create an environment where trainees can take risks, stretch beyond their comfort zones, and grow into the physicians they are capable of becoming.

Recovery helped me recognize my own wounds, and in doing so, taught me how to care for others and teach with greater humility and humanity. By tending to my own inner landscape, I learned how to create safer spaces for patients and trainees to bring their full selves into the room.

That, to me, is psychological safety and trauma-informed care in practice.

Systemic Change

If trauma-informed care is to be more than an individual virtue or bedside skill, it must be intentionally embedded into the systems in which we practice. Systemic change begins with a fundamental acknowledgment that trauma isn't an exception in healthcare. It's pervasive. Patients arrive carrying histories of violence, loss, discrimination, medical harm, and chronic stress. Clinicians, too, accumulate trauma through repeated exposure to suffering, high-stakes decision-making, moral injury, and unsafe working conditions. When systems fail to recognize this reality, they often recreate the very dynamics that define traumatic experience, including powerlessness, loss of agency, silencing, unpredictability, and fear. This happens despite the best intentions of the people working within them.

A truly trauma-informed system would redesign care processes to restore agency wherever possible. Consent would be treated as an ongoing conversation rather than a single signature or verbal checkpoint, with clinicians trained and supported to pause, check in, and adapt throughout an encounter. Protocols would be flexible enough to offer alternatives to invasive exams when clinically appropriate, to slow down when patients show signs of distress, and to honor a patient's right to say no without penalty or judgment. Requests for provider gender preference would be normalized rather than treated as inconvenient, and systems would develop thoughtful mechanisms such as standardized trauma summaries or discreet chart indicators to reduce the need for patients to disclose painful histories repeatedly

Leaders would be required to receive training in trauma-aware management as well. Such training begins with understanding that leadership is never neutral. In healthcare, authority figures do more than convey information. They regulate nervous systems. For individuals with trauma histories, power, tone, and unpredictability have the potential to recreate the conditions of threat and helplessness that define traumatic experience.

Power is especially potent in medical hierarchies, where leaders influence evaluations, schedules, opportunities, and careers. A comment meant as casual guidance can land as judgment, and public correction can feel like humiliation. Trauma-aware leaders recognize that impact matters more than intent and consistently stay curious about how their words will be received, given the imbalance of power.

Trauma-informed systems would also turn their attention inward, recognizing that clinician trauma isn't a personal weakness but an occupational reality. Instead of pathologizing individual responses to overwhelming environments, these systems would approach provider distress with curiosity and compassion. Protected time and space for reflection, debriefing, and emotional processing would be built into clinical workflows rather than offered only after catastrophic events.

Importantly, trauma-informed systems would explicitly acknowledge that substance use, depression, anxiety, and burnout among clinicians are *not* moral failings or professionalism lapses. Sometimes they are signals of injury within the system itself. By shifting the question from, *"What's wrong with this provider?"* to *"What has this provider been carrying, and how have we contributed?"* institutions would begin to dismantle cultures of silence that endanger both clinicians and patients.

Finally, trauma-informed systemic change requires reexamining the structural drivers of harm. Staffing models, documentation, productivity metrics, and scheduling practices must be evaluated for their impact on mental health. Trauma-aware leadership asks different questions, like, *"Is this sustainable? Does this create a safe environment for the people delivering care?"* When productivity demands consistently override basic needs for rest, connection, and recovery, trauma isn't an unintended side effect. It's a predictable outcome.

Trauma-informed systemic change asks medicine to confront a difficult truth: we cannot build healing environments based on fear, control, and exhaustion and expect compassion to endure. When systems intentionally prioritize dignity, shared power, and psychological safety for patients and clinicians alike, trauma-informed care becomes the default rather than the exception.

Final Thoughts

When I finally came out, not just as a gay man, but as someone in recovery and someone with trauma, something relaxed within me. I stopped pretending and started connecting. I stopped trying to earn my place and started trusting that I belonged. Not surprisingly, I became a better doctor. I became more present and more human.

Trauma-informed care doesn't just heal our patients. It heals us, too. It asks us to slow down, stay curious, and remember that every person, ourselves included, has a story that shapes how they show up in the world. When we ask, "*What happened to you?*" and then turn it inward to say, "*What happened to me?*" we begin to create healthcare systems that honor not just physical illness, but the entire soul.

REFLECTION QUESTIONS

1. Do you have any childhood trauma that affects how you show up at work?
2. Have you ever judged a patient before understanding their story? What assumptions did you make?

3. What is one way you can bring more compassion to yourself this week?
4. Do you believe that acknowledging your own pain could make you a better clinician? Why or why not?

COMMUNITY & SERVICE

There were nine of us. Eight women and me, matched into the same residency program. Strangers at first, we became teammates, then something more like family. On paper, we were just another class of OBGYN residents. But beneath the surface, we were a mosaic of lived experience, each of us carrying things we didn't talk about in morning sign-out or during rounds. Things that shaped the way we practiced medicine, and the way we held each other through it.

Medical training is brutal for everyone; nurses, doctors, midlevel providers—you name it. That's not news. But what no one prepares you for is how much life keeps happening outside the hospital walls, be it illness, grief, loss, or addiction. No one realizes how those outside influences can seep into your body as you're trying to learn how to care for other people's lives. That was our reality.

Three of us had family members diagnosed with cancer (one of whom passed away during our training). Another received the devastating news that a parent had died by suicide.

Another faced a complicated pregnancy of her own while caring for others, haunted by the same fears she'd seen in so many of her patients. Another missed milestones of her teenage children as they were growing up. And then there was me, trying to fight the battle against addiction.

Through grief and relapse, death and despair, we showed up for each other in the ways that mattered most. When one of us was falling apart, the others leaned in. We covered shifts without asking why. We checked in on one another. We sat in call rooms and cried together. We made each other laugh in ways only people who've seen too much can. It was the quiet, relentless work of love, a kind of mutual tending. We didn't need to fix each other. We just needed to be there for one another. And we were.

My residency class taught me more about medicine than any textbook or lecture ever could. They showed me how to sit beside someone who is suffering without looking away. Even when I was barely holding it together myself, I learned how to say, "I've got you" to someone else. I discovered what it means to keep showing up—not out of obligation, but because I am tethered to something larger than myself. Community.

The truth is, none of us would have made it through on our own. We needed each other in the most honest, human ways. And it wasn't resilience that got us through. It was grace. It was solidarity. It was the radical act of choosing not to let each other go.

Years later, I still carry each of them with me. In every delivery room, every difficult conversation, every moment I feel like I don't belong, I remember the faces of eight women who reminded me, over and over again, that I do belong. My co-residents didn't just help me survive residency; they helped me thrive. They helped me find my way back to myself.

Community & Service in Recovery

They say the opposite of addiction is connection. Connection to people. To purpose. To community.

That's why mutual support meetings, whether they're 12-step programs or any form of peer-led gathering, are not just helpful; they are essential to healing. In those rooms, recovery begins with eye contact and nods of recognition rather than jumping right into instruction. It starts with hearing someone else say the thing you were too ashamed to say out loud. You listen, and you realize, maybe for the first time, that you are not alone.

I recently came across a list of the top public health achievements of the twentieth century: penicillin, vaccines, tobacco cessation, and seat belts. All worthy inclusions. But I was struck by a glaring omission. There was no mention of mutual support communities for addiction. And yet, in my opinion, they deserve to be near the top of that list.

Because if we, as a society, truly understood the number of lives saved every single day in church basements, community centers, and on video-conference screens around the world, we'd realize this is nothing short of a miracle. These groups aren't funded by governments or managed by professionals. They don't rely on clinics or credentials. They rely on people. These are people who've been to the brink, and who are now reaching back to pull others away from the edge.

We continue to underestimate addiction's death toll. Rarely does a death certificate read "addiction" as the cause of death. Instead, it says "heart failure," "stroke," "respiratory arrest," "sepsis," "cancer," "suicide," "vehicular trauma," "failure to thrive." But trace those conditions back, and time and time again you'll find a common thread: Addiction. Often untreated, unseen, or actively stigmatized, it remains the root cause beneath so many of the diseases we label as primary.

So, when you ask what saves lives from addiction, the answer goes beyond detox units or buprenorphine prescriptions. It goes beyond therapy. Therapy helps...but community sustains. Above all, lives are saved through the unconditional, radically inclusive connection forged in the rooms of recovery.

These rooms reflect every demographic and every background. They're filled with Republicans, Democrats, Christians, Muslims, atheists, Black, white, Asian, Latino, rich, poor, housed, unhoused, queer, trans, and non-binary. Addiction doesn't discriminate, and neither does recovery. For one sacred hour, all of those differences fade. You sit in a circle, and you share a common truth: your pain is my pain. Your story is mine, too.

When I first entered recovery, I felt like I had two separate lives. One was the professional, polished doctor who excelled at his work. The other was the person who had spiraled in silence, numbed with substances, and was now trying to piece together a life without them. These lives felt irreconcilable. I didn't know where I belonged.

At traditional 12-step meetings, I found relief, but I also found myself holding back. I was afraid someone might recognize me or ask what I did for work. I was afraid that even in a room full of people who understood addiction, they might not understand the shame of being a physician who couldn't keep it all together. I thought no one else would understand the crushing fear of licensure boards and the impossible pressure to return to work like nothing had happened.

And then I was introduced to a closed 12-step meeting for healthcare professionals. It was a room full of physicians, nurses, dentists, and therapists, all of whom understood the unbearable tension of holding others' pain while avoiding their own. For the first time, I didn't have to explain the impossible expectations. They just got it.

I remember the first meeting I attended. Someone shared about returning to work after treatment and being terrified they'd be exposed. Another shared about the death of a patient and how it triggered a relapse. Someone else talked about having to sit in front of their hospital credentialing committee and tell the truth for the first time.

I didn't say a word at that meeting. But I silently cried the whole time, because finally, I felt like I had found my people.

Later that week, someone from the group reached out to me to check in, and one week later, that man became my sponsor. A well-respected emergency medicine doctor, he had been sober for nearly 8 years at the time and had rebuilt a life in recovery that was honest, joyful, and deeply connected. "It's my turn to help someone else," he told me. "This is how I stay sober."

Not only had I found a community where I belonged, but for the first time, I understood that being part of a community also means paying it forward. It means serving others and giving them the gift of recovery by sharing my own story.

Over the months that followed, I found my rhythm. I started attending a weekly 'queer physicians in recovery' meeting where I met others whose identities were just as layered and complex as mine. We didn't have to explain our queerness, our professional pressures, or our shame. It was all allowed. All welcomed.

There's a kind of healing that happens when you hear someone else speak the words you've never dared to say aloud. When you laugh at something that once only made you cry. When someone says, "Me too," and you finally believe you're not broken, just human. That's what these meetings have done for me.

I've since attended national recovery conferences for medical professionals. I've sat in banquet halls filled with hundreds of healthcare professionals in recovery, all of us reclaiming our lives and our profession through honesty and community. I've heard stories of redemption that would make your heart burst. I've seen people weep with gratitude and shake with fear.

Every one of them is paying it forward. They're sponsoring newcomers to recovery. They're leading meetings. They're advocating for better monitoring systems, safer spaces, and more compassionate care. They're sharing their stories to invite. To say, "Come sit with us. There's room for you here."

And now, slowly, I am learning to do the same. When I can, I speak. I take phone calls from newcomers and stay after meetings to clean up chairs. Sometimes I text someone just to say I'm thinking of them. It's nothing fancy, yet it means everything. Giving back to my community is how I stay sober and whole.

The Lack of Community in Healthcare

Contrast this environment with modern-day medical culture. We talk endlessly about multidisciplinary teams and the value of collaboration. We write "teamwork" into our mission statements and value "interpersonal skills" in prospective job applicants. But the system is designed to be a hierarchy rather than a true community of equals. I've worked in spaces where the clinicians were just a collection of professionals who passed each other in the hallway. We shared a workspace, but not our lives.

Yes, we have colleagues. But how often do we pause to see them, to notice the stories they carry. Do we know who lost a parent last year? Who is battling depression in silence? Who is navigating a divorce, caring for a chronically ill child, or feeling like an imposter every time they scrub into the OR? Sometimes, in our effort to appear composed, perform well, and survive our shifts, these lives slip by unnoticed. And yet, noticing them, even in small ways, is where connection and understanding begin.

In most hospitals, the physical space reflects the emotional landscape. Attendings are in one room, residents are in another, and nurses are at a separate station. The staff is divided by titles. Notes are passed through EMR messages. People page each other and send texts. But they often don't have time to sit down face-to-face and connect. Add in post-pandemic hybrid work models where providers can treat patients from their living rooms, and they become even more isolated from their teams.

So, how do we deliver compassionate, coordinated care when there are so many obstacles to connection that must be overcome first? How do we build trust with patients if we haven't practiced trust among ourselves? How do we retain clinicians if they never feel truly known?

Burnout is rampant. Suicide among physicians remains devastatingly high. Substance use disorders often go unnoticed in our peers. These patterns force us to ask why and what we can do to change them. Maybe the answer isn't more wellness lectures. Maybe, just maybe, the answer is what recovery taught me years ago: connection, community, and service.

It is my opinion that when we talk about "service" in healthcare, what we are often doing is giving another name to exploitation. The medical culture valorizes overwork and self-sacrifice, and perhaps our good intentions allow us to mistake martyrdom for meaning.

The concept of service, as I understand it through the lens of recovery, is radically different. It's not about being the best, the fastest, or the most altruistic. It's about showing up in quiet, consistent ways for the people who walk this path beside you, especially when they are struggling.

So, what if we brought the ethic of recovery into our departments, hospitals, and academic communities? What if service meant checking in on the intern who looks like they haven't slept? What if it meant offering to co-write that manuscript because someone's drowning? What if it meant texting a colleague to say, "I'm thinking of you. I'm here if you ever want to talk."

Sometimes, we hold back from service because we think we have nothing to give. This is especially true if we don't have it all together in our own personal lives. But recovery has taught me that service isn't something we wait to do until we're fully healed. It's often how the healing happens.

Just as addiction is fueled by disconnection, the antidote to burnout also lies in connection. Because only when we feel safe with one another can we ask for help. Practicing vulnerability in small moments paves the way for us to rely on one another in big ones. And when we are truly known for who we are rather than what we produce, we discover a sense of belonging deep enough to carry us through.

Into Practice

When I stepped into my first leadership role, I was shocked by the sheer volume of complaints that came across my desk. Staff members were frustrated with trainees, and the trainees were upset with staff. Most of the issues stemmed from communication breakdowns, and, as we know, communication failures are among the leading contributors to medical error. But beneath the surface, it became clear these weren't just problems of how people talked to each other. The deeper issue was how disconnected people had become. Our teams didn't know each other. There was no sense of community in our clinical space.

The physical layout of our hospital didn't help. Registration staff sat behind closed doors. Triage nurses were in one area, midlevels and residents in another. L&D nurses had their own area, and some were even sitting all alone at single computer workstations scattered across our floor. Attendings also had their own separate rooms, and Maternal Fetal Medicine was tucked away in the back. Most of our communication happened over the phone, and often without even using names. It's no wonder we struggled to build trust! The fragmentation was built into our structure. And in this new era of medicine, with many trainees more fluent in digital communication than in face-to-face interaction, those barriers are even harder to overcome.

But my experience in recovery taught me the immeasurable value of human interaction. It cannot be said enough that community saves lives. It certainly saved mine. I am in no small part alive and sober today because I belong to a group of people who show up for me and keep me accountable. That knowledge shapes the way I practice medicine. I now see building community in healthcare as essential to our survival. Everyone in the ecosystem—residents, nurses, midwives, techs, staff, security—deserves to feel seen and valued.

So, I try to bring these principles into my day-to-day clinical work by creating small but meaningful daily rituals that ground our teams. Whether it's starting a shift with a moment of gratitude or pausing to debrief after a tough case, these rituals create space for connection and healing. I also pay close attention to the language I use with my teams. I lean on phrases that reflect the humility and compassion I've learned in recovery, like "We're learning together" or "Thank you for teaching me that." My goal is to reinforce honesty, curiosity, and psychological safety in everything I say and do.

Celebrating human moments has also become a priority for me. Clinical work can be relentless, but taking time to acknowledge birthdays, small wins, or a particularly beautiful patient interaction can shift the energy on the floor. Those pauses matter, and they remind us why we're here. So does modeling vulnerability. Recovery taught me that change starts when someone is brave enough to go first. When I speak about my anxiety, my struggles in training, and my journey with addiction (appropriately and transparently), it opens the door for others to do the same. Culture change can only happen when leaders lead differently.

Acts of service don't have to be grand to be powerful. Sometimes, it's bringing in coffee for the team on a tough morning. Sometimes it's texting someone after a long shift to say, "You were incredible today." Sometimes it's picking up the phone when a colleague across the country is struggling and needs to know they're not alone.

Service also means mentoring. When I mentor someone, I don't just offer guidance. I share my own missteps and stay open to learning from my mentees in return. Recovery taught me that mentorship is mutual growth, and I carry that belief into every conversation with residents and medical students.

There are also times when service means advocating outside the clinical space. I write, speak, and push for systemic change, even when it's uncomfortable. I share my recovery journey in professional forums, despite being told that it's risky to do so, because transparency is a form of service, too. Every time I tell the truth about how close I came to walking away from medicine, and how recovery gave me a second chance, I create space for someone else to stay.

And of course, I carry this spirit into my patient care. Sometimes, I sit across from a patient battling addiction, and I can feel the wall between us: the shame, the fear, the sense that they're about to be judged. When it feels right, I say, "I'm in recovery. I get it." That moment of shared humanity allows their guard to come down. They trust me. They come back because they see someone who's been where they are and who made it through.

In that moment, we're not just doctor and patient. We're two people sharing a path, however briefly. That's community, too. A circle of belonging that says, "You matter. You're not alone. You're safe here."

Healing is relational. Communities that thrive aren't the ones that never fracture. They are the ones that know how to repair. That kind of repair only happens when we share commitments out loud and live them consistently. In recovery, we have the Twelve Steps. In medicine, I dream of teams that create their own shared values: to speak truthfully, own mistakes, support each other, prioritize people over productivity, and hold each other accountable with kindness. These aren't pipe dreams. They're possible, but only if we're willing to do the work.

That work starts with service. Showing up for others. Listening. Offering grace. And remembering that, just like recovery, medicine is not a solo journey. We get better together. Always.

Systemic Change

Systemic change, when viewed through the lens of community and service, requires medicine to fundamentally rethink how we define professionalism, productivity, and belonging. It may feel impossible to change institutions that have been organized around hierarchy and individual performance for so long. But it's not. A system oriented toward community would acknowledge that healthcare isn't sustained by lone heroes but by interconnected people.

At a structural level, this means intentionally designing environments that foster relationships rather than fragmentation. Physical spaces matter. When teams are separated by walls, locked doors, and isolated workstations, disconnection becomes the default. Systemic change would prioritize shared spaces where interdisciplinary teams can gather, debrief, and relate as humans, not just roles. It would also challenge the rigid silos that divide attendings from residents, nurses from physicians, and clinical staff from non-clinical staff. Community cannot grow in environments where power differentials are constantly reinforced and humanity is compartmentalized.

A community-centered system would also fundamentally rethink how it responds to clinician suffering. Instead of treating grief, addiction, depression, burnout, or moral injury as individual weaknesses to be hidden, institutions would make support visible, relational, and non-punitive. In such systems, distress is viewed as an expected human response to difficult work. With this understanding, the goal shifts from containing liability to restoring connection.

Central to this shift is the integration of peer-led support groups into the fabric of healthcare organizations. These are clinician-driven spaces grounded in shared lived experience, modeled after recovery communities where people heal by being seen. In these settings, clinicians don't retreat behind roles or titles. They gather together as human beings who have lost patients, made mistakes, been afraid, felt overwhelmed, or sometimes even questioned whether they can keep going.

For these groups to succeed at a systems level, institutions must protect their autonomy while actively supporting their existence. This means providing physical space, protected time, and logistical resources without exerting control over content or participation. Leadership endorsement matters, but ownership must remain with peers. Institutions can identify and train facilitators drawn from within the clinician community, particularly those with lived experience of recovery, burnout, or moral injury. Training should focus not on fixing or advising, but on listening, boundary-setting, and trauma-informed group facilitation.

Importantly, peer support groups should be diverse in form and accessible across roles and identities. Some providers may benefit from general peer support, while others may need affinity-based spaces. This could include groups for trainees, nurses, physicians, LGBTQ+ clinicians, clinicians in recovery, or those involved in adverse events. Offering multiple entry points acknowledges that community can take many different forms and may make these spaces feel more accessible.

Peer-led support also serves a critical preventive function. By creating regular spaces for reflection and connection, these groups allow distress to be named early, before it escalates into crisis, impairment, or departure from the profession. They reduce isolation and counter shame, while providing a corrective experience to the culture of silence that pervades healthcare.

Over time, they can shift institutional norms, making it more acceptable to ask for help when needed.

Finally, a system grounded in community would require a redefinition of leadership itself. Leaders would be selected and rewarded for their capacity to cultivate trust, repair harm, and foster a genuine sense of belonging, as well as for their operational efficiency. This kind of leadership is less about control and more about stewardship. It requires the humility to listen and the willingness to be accountable when harm occurs. Leaders in community-centered systems aren't distant overseers; they are visible participants in the shared life of the department.

At a practical level, this shift would be reflected in how departmental initiatives are designed and carried out. Community-building would be woven into the everyday rhythms of work. Meetings, in particular, would be recognized as powerful cultural spaces. Instead of focusing exclusively on dashboards, deficits, and deliverables, meetings would intentionally make room for meaning. This could include brief check-ins that invite people to name how they are arriving to the space, acknowledgments of recent challenges or losses, or moments of gratitude that recognize unseen labor. These practices don't require excessive time; they require intention. Even a few minutes dedicated to human connection can fundamentally shift how safe and collaborative a room feels.

When leadership is practiced this way, community ceases to be an abstract ideal and becomes a lived experience that allows people to support one another more honestly.

Final Thoughts

In recovery, community saves lives by replacing isolation with connection and shame with shared humanity. Medicine doesn't need to reinvent this truth; it needs to remember it. If we want to stem burnout, reduce harm, and retain clinicians who still believe in the soul of this work, we must build systems that make connection the norm. Community is a structural necessity. And service, when practiced collectively and compassionately amongst ourselves, is how community endures.

REFLECTION QUESTIONS

1. When was the last time you felt truly seen and supported by someone you work with? What made that moment meaningful?
2. Is there a colleague you've been holding at arm's length who might be carrying something heavy you don't know about?
3. What barriers prevent deeper connection in your work environment? How might you start to shift one of them?
4. In what ways can you contribute to a sense of community among your team?

GRATITUDE

I was an intern, still learning how to stand upright in my scrubs, let alone how to deliver a baby with confidence. I felt like a fish out of water in obstetrics, desperate to absorb every detail, every clinical nuance, every skill I could get my hands on. I was rotating at a small community hospital just outside Minneapolis. There was nothing particularly remarkable about the place. It served a largely healthy, upper-middle-class population. Quiet. Predictable. A good place to learn the basics.

Years later, out of all the complex deliveries and the clinical emergencies I've seen, I still hold on to one simple thing I witnessed during my rotation at this hospital.

It happened after a calm and uneventful birth for a healthy mom and baby. We were wrapping up, counseling the patient on what to expect next, and ready to move on. But before we left the room, my attending turned to the new mother and gently said,

"Thank you for letting us take care of you today. Thank you for letting us be part of your birth."

The patient and her partner looked up and smiled. "Of course," they replied. "Thank you, too."

It was such a small exchange, yet it had a huge impact on me. Up until that point, I had assumed gratitude was something patients were supposed to express. "Thank you, Doctor," was a phrase I heard often. But this was different. This was gratitude in reverse.

In that moment, I stopped thinking about what I needed to perfect and started remembering what a privilege it is to do this work. People let us into their most vulnerable moments: birth, illness, uncertainty, grief. They hand us their bodies, their stories, and their hopes. And we're expected to hold all of it with care.

That day, I realized something that I'll carry with me for the rest of my career. I don't just provide care. I get to be a part of something sacred. I get to show up. I get to be trusted. I get to serve. And for that, I am deeply grateful. Gratitude doesn't erase the pain or pressure of this work. It does reframe it, however. And it reminds us, on even the hardest days, that we're part of something that matters.

Gratitude in Recovery

Gratitude is so much more than saying "thank you." It's a conscious practice of noticing, pausing, appreciating, and allowing what is, rather than constantly chasing what is not. It's the daily decision to reframe "not enough" into "what a gift."

In addiction, I was constantly chasing more—more drugs, more alcohol, more highs, more money, more attention, more achievement. Beneath that chase lived a belief I never said aloud but felt deep in my bones: *I am not enough.*

I remember being a third-year resident constantly living outside the present moment. Irritation colored everything about my daily life, from my workload to my supervisors to my partner. I couldn't sit still. My mind was always scanning for the next opportunity to stand out and get recognition. To feel important. More money, more accolades, nicer possessions, and a bigger home all felt essential to achieving a better life. What I really wanted most was validation.

And then, I got sick.

Addiction, which had been quietly brewing beneath my ambition, broke the surface. I spiraled and began using more. Everything I'd worked so hard for began slipping through my fingers.

Looking back, I see now that my insatiable hunger for more was about disconnection. I couldn't feel grateful for the life in front of me because I was too blinded by what I thought was missing. My sense of worth was entirely based on accolades and superficial things. It wasn't until I entered recovery that I began to understand the power of gratitude.

In early recovery, the idea of gratitude felt impossible. I was ashamed and afraid. My brain wasn't wired to see the good. But slowly, as I listened to others share what they were grateful for (sunlight through a window, a call from a friend, one more day sober), I began to see what was still available to me.

Gratitude requires intentionality. Some days it's hard to be grateful. Really hard. But even on those days, I've learned

I can find something. A moment of laughter. A clear mind. The chance to show up for someone else. Gratitude isn't about pretending everything is okay. It's about noticing that even when things are hard, there is still beauty here. There is still enough.

In recovery, we often talk about what leads people back to substance use. The answers are predictable: resentment, entitlement, comparison, shame. Gratitude is the opposite of all those things. It's the cure.

Gratitude dissolves resentment by shifting our focus from what we lack to what we have. In doing so, it interrupts entitlement by reminding us that nothing is promised and everything is a gift. It calms comparison by allowing us to celebrate our own unique path, and it neutralizes shame by showing us that we are already worthy, already enough.

If that's not medicine, I don't know what is.

Into Practice

Before entering recovery, my work in medicine felt heavy with obligation. Charting. Rounding. Answering pages. Teaching. Meetings. Counseling the same patient for the fifth time. Finishing administrative work long after my shift had ended. My days felt reactive, dictated by endless demands, and I moved through them with a constant sense of scarcity; there was never enough time or support. Never enough room to breathe.

Over time, my work became transactional. I was burned out, disconnected, and quietly bitter.

Recovery steadily changed that. As I began practicing gratitude in my personal life, I noticed how profoundly it shifted my outlook. So, I wondered what might happen if I brought that same practice into medicine. What if I stopped framing my work as a list of obligations and started seeing it as a series of opportunities? I began paying attention to the moments when my inner dialogue said, "I have to," and I practiced gently rewriting them as "I get to."

I noticed the shift immediately. Showing up for my shift no longer felt like an obligation. It felt like I was being invited into someone's story. Discharge paperwork became the chance to help someone go home. Precepting a student turned into an opportunity to help shape the future of medicine. Explaining a diagnosis for the third time became a way to bring clarity during a frightening moment. Answering pages all night meant being trusted to help people when they needed it most. When I had to work another holiday, it became a way to offer comfort to those who couldn't be home. Even conversations with frustrated family members became opportunities to be a bridge between fear and understanding.

As I write this chapter, I'm deeply aware of how many people make it possible for me to show up fully. I've been extraordinarily lucky to work alongside coworkers who are kind, funny, compassionate, and deeply dedicated. They have carried me through hard days, hard months, and some of the most vulnerable moments of my recovery. They welcomed me back after a leave of absence without judgment and helped dissolve shame through quiet acts of support.

I am also profoundly grateful for the students and residents who allow me to be their teacher. It still amazes me that I get to help shape the next generation of physicians. Teaching isn't something I take lightly. It's an honor and one that gives far more back than it asks. The curiosity, intelligence, and insight of my students continually remind me that learning is lifelong and reciprocal.

And then there are the multidisciplinary teams (nurses, midlevel providers, residents, anesthesiologists, consultants) who show up every day ready to do the impossible together. We laugh together. We grieve together. We save lives together. On the hardest days, I am grateful beyond words to work alongside people I trust when the stakes are highest.

One case, in particular, lives with me. A patient arrived at the triage unit late one night with vaginal bleeding and contractions in the third trimester. Her name was Fernanda. She had received most of her care outside the country, and her records were limited. A language barrier made gathering her history challenging, but we learned she had a history of preeclampsia and three prior cesarean deliveries.

Initially, Fernanda appeared stable. Her labs were reassuring. But as we continued monitoring, her blood pressure climbed, and the fetal heart rate began dropping with contractions. Given her surgical history, I worried about placenta accreta, which is a condition in which the placenta grows deeply into the wall of the uterus and doesn't detach normally after birth. Thankfully, our ultrasound images didn't show any overtly concerning features for abnormal placentation. Taken together, the picture pointed toward placental abruption, and we moved quickly to the operating room.

From the moment we entered the abdomen, I knew we were in trouble. There was dense scar tissue and significant bleeding. After painstaking dissection, we delivered the baby. The placenta appeared to be separating easily, and, for a brief moment, I exhaled. But then the uterus began hemorrhaging catastrophically. As we worked, I immediately understood that we were facing an undiagnosed placenta accreta, adhered deeply and invisibly.

Blood loss was massive. The room transformed instantly. Nurses prepared for an emergency hysterectomy. Anesthesia transfused blood without pause. My co-attending and fellow were scrubbed in before I could ask. The gynecologic oncologist was already on her way to help with the complicated surgery. Eight units of blood later, we removed the uterus. The bleeding stopped, and Fernanda survived. She recovered fully.

At the end of that case, I was physically depleted but also overwhelmed with gratitude. An undiagnosed accreta is one of the most frightening scenarios in obstetrics. Things could have gone very differently. But because of that team, because of their skill, trust, and teamwork, our patient lived. A mother got to go home and watch her baby boy grow up.

I return to that case often, especially on quiet, mundane days. It reminds me why gratitude matters, and what I have to be grateful for. Ultimately, I've found that if I don't practice gratitude, I start to lose my sense of meaning, and that loss is the true root of burnout. But gratitude reminds me why I'm here and helps me stay grounded even in the most challenging circumstances.

One way I ground myself in gratitude is by beginning my day with intention. On my way into the hospital, I ask myself, "What am I thankful for right now?" Some days, it's something big, like being healthy or having the ability to serve. Other days, it's as simple as a warm cup of coffee or an easy commute to work.

At the end of the day, I also take time to reflect. I ask myself, "What surprised me today? What moved me?" These reflections remind me that there's always something that touches me. Maybe a patient's story, a learner's insight, or an unexpected moment of connection. That's how I find meaning in the midst of chaos—by remembering the moments that mattered.

With my teams, I've started incorporating gratitude into our shared spaces. During huddles or debriefs, I'll invite people to share one thing they're grateful for from the shift. It doesn't have to be anything profound. Sometimes it's, "I'm grateful for how everyone jumped in during that delivery," or "Someone brought snacks today, and it made my whole afternoon." These moments shift our dynamic from transactional to relational. They remind us that we aren't just getting through, we're doing it together.

Gratitude has also reshaped how I interact with patients. I no longer wait to be thanked; instead, I try to thank them. I say things like, "Thank you for trusting me today," or "It's an honor to care for you." These words matter. They soften the room, they humanize both of us, and they remind me that this work is a privilege.

I also keep a gratitude list. Whether in a notebook or a note on my phone, I jot down three things at the end of the day that made me smile, made me think, or made me feel connected. Especially during challenging seasons, this practice keeps me grounded. It reorients me back to purpose.

Gratitude also builds trust among colleagues. A sincere "thank you" goes a long way. It communicates: *I see you. You matter. You're not alone in this.* I say it often and mean it. "Thank you for your help earlier. You handled that really well," or "I learned something from you today."

These words don't cost anything. But their impact can be profound, especially in high-stress environments where validation is scarce.

Systemic Change

If we want to bring gratitude into our clinical spaces, we must consider building it into the architecture of how healthcare teams function. Systemic gratitude is a disciplined practice of noticing and naming what is working, who is carrying the work, and which moments deserve to be honored. In environments that are trained to scan for risk, error, and deficit, gratitude functions as a corrective lens that restores balance. Practically, this means making gratitude a default part of team rituals.

One of the simplest and most powerful ways to do this is to normalize brief, specific words of gratitude in team huddles. Imagine if every Labor & Delivery huddle began with a 30-second round of appreciation: one concrete action that made a difference, one assist that mattered, or one small win worth naming. We don't want vague affirmations like "great job, everyone," but precise acknowledgments such as, "Thank you for catching that subtle tracing change early." "Thank you for staying late to restock the hemorrhage cart." "Thank you for translating calmly when the room felt chaotic." These micro-acknowledgments take less than two minutes, yet they meaningfully shift the emotional climate of a unit. They help teams feel seen by reinforcing high-value behaviors. It reminds people that their work matters.

Gratitude also needs a place in our operational systems. Many hospitals have sophisticated pathways for reporting errors, near misses, and adverse events. But almost none have an equally frictionless way to document what goes right. A gratitude-informed system would create one. This might take the form of a simple, EMR-adjacent "kudos" tool or a QR code posted in staff areas, allowing anyone—nurses, residents, attendings, transport staff, environmental services—to send a short, specific note of appreciation that is routed to the individual and shared with their supervisor. Practices like these are structural counterweights to a culture that tracks only failure. When gratitude is documented, it becomes visible. When it is visible, it becomes legitimate.

Over time, these acknowledgments can be integrated into performance conversations, promotion considerations, and leadership development. Patterns of gratitude reveal who reliably shows up for others, who communicates well under pressure, and who quietly stabilizes the team during crises. In this way, systemic gratitude helps organizations reward the behaviors that actually improve safety and patient experience, rather than only highlighting individual productivity or technical prowess.

Another practical shift involves redesigning debriefing practices. In a gratitude-informed system, debriefs wouldn't focus solely on what went wrong or what needs fixing. Instead, they would follow a balanced structure: *What happened clinically? What did we learn?* And critically, *who helped us get through it?* Naming contributions during debriefs does more than boost morale; it reinforces behaviors that prevent harm and strengthens team cohesion in the aftermath of high-stress events.

Finally, systemic gratitude must intentionally flow down the hierarchy because that's where medicine most often fractures. Leaders can operationalize this by adopting a rule of visible appreciation, one specific thank-you each day directed toward someone with less formal power. These moments matter because gratitude is a form of equity; it redistributes dignity. It makes invisible labor visible and reminds everyone that safe, compassionate care is a collective achievement, not an individual performance.

When gratitude is built into systems, it becomes a stabilizing force that sustains teams, strengthens trust, and quietly protects the humanity of the people doing the work.

Final Thoughts

Gratitude isn't about denying the hard parts of medicine. It's about remembering what makes it worthwhile. It's not a fix for the broken system, but it *is* a way to stay whole within the system as we work to improve it. For me, gratitude is a recovery principle that helps me show up with heart, again and again.

When I practice gratitude, it gives others permission to do the same. And slowly, one moment of gratitude at a time, it changes the feel of a room, reminding us that even amid the chaos, we are still connected, still learning, still alive. That, in itself, is something to be grateful for.

Reflection Questions

1. What are three things you are grateful for today?
2. When was the last time you expressed gratitude to a colleague? How did it feel?
3. When have you received gratitude from someone else in a way that really stuck with you? What made it meaningful?
4. Which of the practices listed above can you commit to practicing in the workplace tomorrow?

INTEGRITY

It was 3:17 a.m. on Labor & Delivery, that quiet hour of the night when the unit looks calm on paper but never truly feels at rest. The board was mostly green. There were no active hemorrhages. No emergent cesareans. No alarms sounding. By every operational metric, this should have been a lull. And yet my body told a different story. I was seated at a computer in my call room, finishing notes. My shoulders felt tight as my eyes flicked between the screen and the clock, calculating how much sleep I might get if nothing else happened. Even in stillness, the pace of medicine lived inside me.

Then I received a page. A patient's name flashed on the screen. Emily was a first-time mother who had been admitted to the hospital in early labor and was feeling anxious. The note read: "*requests to speak with MD again.*"

I hesitated. I had already been in her room twice. I explained the plan. I reviewed expectations. I answered her questions carefully, methodically, and kindly. The resident was just there as well. Part of me wanted to send the resident back with reassurance, a calm voice, and a familiar script. It would be just enough of a delay to buy me time to finish charting and, maybe, lie down.

Still, something inside me tightened. I recognized the feeling immediately, the quiet internal friction that shows up when my values and my impulses drift apart. Because I knew what she was really asking for was not more information. She was asking for safety. For permission to be uncertain. For someone to sit with her fear rather than manage it away. She was asking to be seen.

I paused and took a breath. Closing the chart, I walked back into her room. The lights were dim, and Emily was lying in bed, eyes wide, hands resting tensely on her abdomen. Instead of standing at the bedside, I pulled up a chair and sat down so we were at eye level. The simple act of sitting felt like a small rebellion against the general pace of L&D. I softened my voice and asked, "How can I help? Tell me what you're most worried about right now."

Emily's shoulders dropped almost immediately. The words came slowly at first, then all at once. She was afraid of losing control, of the unpredictability of labor. She was afraid of the pain, and at the same time, afraid of how an epidural would affect her labor progress. She was worried about every decision and if it was the right one. She was concerned for her baby's wellbeing and her own. And she was also worried that once things started moving, she would no longer be allowed to pause to ask a question or change her mind. She wasn't asking for answers. She was simply asking for reassurance that she would still have agency when things started to feel overwhelming.

We talked for only a few minutes. I didn't offer anything new medically. The plan didn't change. I simply listened and reflected back what I heard. I reminded her that she was allowed to change her mind, that we would keep checking in, and that she was not alone in this. By the time I stood to leave, Emily's breathing had slowed. The room felt quieter, steadier. So did I.

Nothing about that interaction will ever appear in a quality dashboard. There's no billing code for sitting down and certainly no metric for building trust. And yet I know, viscerally, that if I had chosen efficiency and documentation over being present with the patient, I would have walked away carrying another small fracture inside myself.

That fracture has a name. It's called misalignment. Over time, those fractures accumulate into something corrosive. They harden into moral injury, the psychological and spiritual harm that occurs when we are forced to make choices that erode the core values that brought us into medicine in the first place. Over time, these choices exact a cost, and that cost is our integrity.

Integrity is one of those words that gets tossed around often in medicine, usually in mission statements or policy manuals. But at its core, integrity means that who we say we are and how we behave are in alignment. It means our values, identity, and actions are not at odds. Integrity is about being honest with others and with ourselves.

When we live without integrity, we are disconnected from ourselves, from our purpose, and from the things that matter most.

Integrity in Recovery

I never actually learned what integrity was during medical school. We were taught the basic principles of ethics, but never explicitly what it meant to practice medicine with integrity. We were never asked to make a list of our values or to notice when we felt out of alignment with those values. Therefore, it's not surprising that we as healthcare providers have a difficult time pushing back against moral injury, as many of us don't even understand what it is.

I didn't truly grasp the meaning of integrity until I entered recovery. Before that, I was too busy trying to stay afloat. I didn't take time to reflect on my values because I was too ashamed of who I had become. I broke promise after promise, not just to others, but to myself. I swore I would stop using drugs. I didn't show up for my sister when she was undergoing chemotherapy. I cheated in a relationship. I skipped out on responsibilities at work. I lied. I deceived. I disappeared.

And yet, I had been raised with values. My parents taught me to be honest, kind, and dependable. So every time I acted outside of that, the dissonance grew louder. I knew who I wanted to be, but my actions repeatedly contradicted that image. Shame began to seep into every corner of my life. I felt fragmented, split in two. And when you live like that long enough, you begin to lose sight of who you are entirely.

When I finally entered treatment for my substance use disorder, one of the first things they asked us to do was write a list of our values. I remember staring at a blank page, unsure of what to write. It was as if I had lost the language of who I was. But slowly, as others shared, something stirred inside me. I remembered how I was raised. I thought of the person I used to be and the person I didn't want to be anymore.

From that, my values began to emerge — kindness, honesty, patience, presence, and accountability. Little by little, I reclaimed myself. That's when recovery truly began. When I started living in alignment with my values again. When my actions started to reflect the kind of man I wanted to be, not perfectly, but intentionally, day by day.

The Erosion of Integrity in Medicine

Practicing integrity in healthcare means acting in alignment with one's values. But unlike recovery, where that alignment is celebrated, in medicine, we're often pulled out of integrity in subtle, relentless ways. It's the note you copy forward instead of rewriting because you're already behind. It's the concern you don't raise in a meeting because you're tired and want to end on time. It's the patient you rush because you have a million other things to do. It's the injustice you witness and silently absorb because speaking up feels futile or dangerous.

Each time we compromise, it feels small. But over time, the weight adds up. Imagine picking up a small stone and putting it in your pocket every time you act against your values. Now imagine picking up one of those stones every hour of every shift. Eventually, you are carrying a mountain. Eventually, you are buried beneath gravel, and you cannot breathe for the weight of all the rocks.

That is moral injury. And it shows up in many ways: indifference, dishonesty, ethical compromise, arrogance, entitlement, deflection, distraction, rushed care, condescension, control, rigidity, judgment, assumption, inequity, discrimination, self-interest, silence, avoidance, complicity, bitterness, isolation, competitiveness, to name a few.

Do you recognize any of these in your place of work? In yourself? That's not failure. That's a call to return to your center. We won't always get it right. Integrity is not perfection. It's alignment. Every time we drift from it, we are invited to return.

Into Practice

Just as in recovery, I realized the first step to reclaiming my integrity in medicine was to reconnect with my values. I had to ask myself, "What do I stand for? What matters most? Why did I enter medicine in the first place?" Some of my values have already been mentioned in this book (honesty, surrender, presence, community, safety, etc.), but the list extends far beyond the chapter titles. Below is a list of additional values, what they mean to me, how my experiences in healthcare pull me away from them, and the things I try to do daily to realign myself.

Compassion, for me, is the willingness to remain emotionally present in the face of suffering without hardening or turning away. It's not simply feeling for someone; it's allowing their experience to matter to me, even when I'm tired, overwhelmed, or under pressure to move on. In medicine, compassion is often the first casualty of efficiency, and I feel myself pulled away from compassion when I begin to see patients as tasks to complete rather than people to encounter. To realign, I intentionally slow down in small ways, such as sitting instead of standing, avoiding referencing the electronic medical record during patient encounters, and avoiding looking at my watch. Even brief moments of genuine compassion restore both the patient's sense of safety and my own sense of purpose.

Empathy deepens compassion by asking me to imagine what it feels like to be the person in front of me, rather than simply understanding their condition. It's the capacity to say, without judgment, "That makes sense. I understand." Medicine pulls me away from empathy through repeated exposure to trauma at the workplace and an unspoken expectation to armor myself emotionally. Over time, self-protection can masquerade as professionalism, leaving me efficient but disconnected. I realign with empathy by staying curious about my patients and by reminding myself that a person's behavior may be reflecting fear, grief, or prior harm. When I allow myself to feel with patients rather than manage them, the work becomes human again.

Accountability means taking responsibility not only for my intentions, but for my impact. It asks me to acknowledge when

I have caused harm, missed something, or fallen short, and to commit to repair rather than defend myself. Medicine often encourages blame-shifting and self-protection in high-stakes environments where mistakes feel dangerous. I feel pulled away from accountability when fear of judgment overrides honesty. I realign by pausing when defensiveness arises and asking where repair is needed. I apologize when I rush, follow up when I miscommunicate, and model accountability openly so others feel safe doing the same.

Kindness is expressed through our values in the smallest interactions—through our tone, posture, and choice of words. It is choosing gentleness in environments that often reward hardness. Stress, fatigue, and hierarchy can quickly erode kindness, especially when urgency dominates. I realign by being intentional with my words, particularly when I am tired or frustrated, and by remembering that kindness costs little but carries enormous weight.

Respect is the recognition of inherent dignity in every person, regardless of role, status, or circumstance. It's shown in what I say and in how I listen. Medicine's hierarchies and time pressures can normalize dismissiveness, especially toward those with less power. I realign by trying to address everyone by name, listening without interruption, and intervening when I witness disrespect. Respect builds psychological safety, which is essential for patient care and teaching environments.

Open-mindedness allows me to remain flexible rather than rigid, and responsive rather than defensive. It invites growth by making space for perspectives that differ from my own. As we've discussed, medicine often rewards certainty and discourages change, subtly framing openness as weakness. I realign by actively seeking viewpoints that challenge my assumptions and by reminding myself that evolving understanding is a strength. Open-mindedness keeps integrity alive by allowing alignment to grow rather than stagnate.

Curiosity keeps me engaged rather than cynical. It replaces judgment with interest and assumptions with questions. Burnout narrows curiosity into shortcuts. I realign by asking "Why?" instead of concluding, "This is just how they are." This small adjustment helps me remain interested in people. Thus, curiosity transforms frustration into understanding and keeps my work intellectually and emotionally alive.

Justice asks me to recognize that healthcare doesn't occur in a vacuum, but within systems shaped by inequity. It calls me to notice patterns of harm and take action. Healthcare systems today sometimes encourage neutrality, even when neutrality perpetuates injustice. I realign by speaking up when inequity is visible and by advocating for marginalized patients and trainees.

Courage is choosing alignment over approval. It means speaking up, setting boundaries, and naming truth even when it risks discomfort or conflict. Fear of repercussions can quietly erode courage in medicine. I realign by reminding myself that discomfort is temporary, but misalignment lingers. Courage helps to protect my integrity.

Patience allows me to meet people where they are, rather than where I wish they were. Healing and learning rarely follow linear timelines, yet medicine rewards speed and resolution. I realign by slowing my speech, allowing silence, and respecting different paces of understanding and change. I practice patience daily with colleagues, trainees, and those I care for.

Equality reminds me that every person deserves dignity, voice, and care regardless of identity or circumstance. Structural inequities pull medicine away from this ideal daily. I realign by examining my own blind spots, advocating for inclusive care, and challenging systems that perpetuate disparity. Equality requires both awareness and action.

Second chances are central to how I understand healing, both in recovery and in medicine. They reflect my belief that people are more than their worst moment, their poorest decision, or their most visible failure. Medicine often pulls me away from this value by privileging perfection and reputational protection. Errors are remembered longer than efforts, and systems are quick to label rather than rehabilitate. I realign by consciously separating behavior from identity, naming mistakes while also naming potential, and advocating for remediation, support, and reflection whenever possible. Practicing second chances recognizes that growth is iterative and that healing rarely happens without room to try again.

Agency and advocacy are inseparable in how I practice medicine. Agency is the belief that people have the right and the capacity to participate meaningfully in decisions about their bodies, their care, and their lives. Advocacy is what agency requires when systems, power dynamics, or inequities threaten to silence that voice. In medicine, agency is often eroded by time pressure, hierarchy, paternalism, and policies that prioritize efficiency over autonomy. I feel pulled away from these values when care plans are delivered rather than co-created, when patients feel talked at instead of listened to, or when trainees are expected to comply without context. I realign by intentionally inviting patients and learners into shared decision-making, naming options and uncertainties clearly, and asking what matters most to them rather than assuming I know. Advocacy shows up when I use my position to amplify the voices of marginalized people and challenge policies that cause harm.

Systemic Change

If integrity is alignment between what we value and how we practice, then systemic change must make that alignment easier and misalignment less necessary. Right now, too many clinicians are forced into daily "micro-betrayals" of self— rushing when they want to listen, documenting when they'd rather comfort, appeasing hierarchy when they wish they could speak up. A system committed to integrity would start treating these betrayals as predictable outcomes of flawed design. It would build workflows that protect presence, honesty, and relational care as legitimate clinical work.

The most practical place to start is by defining "good care." If the only things that count are throughput, RVUs, discharge times, and note completion, integrity will always lose. *Metrics are not neutral; they quietly define what matters and what gets sacrificed.* These numbers tell us how efficiently we extract labor from clinicians, but they tell us almost nothing about whether care is healing, ethical, or sustainable.

A more integrity-centered system would add metrics that reflect the values we claim to hold. For example, instead of asking how many patients were seen, it would ask whether patients felt seen, heard, and cared for by someone they recognized. Continuity and relational trust become meaningful signals of system health. These metrics might even be early indicators of long-term positive outcomes. When clinicians are given the time and structural support to show up fully, both patients and teams will do better.

Integrity in medicine also requires honesty, and honesty depends on psychological safety. In healthy systems, a higher number of reported near-misses or concerns is not a failure. It's evidence that people feel safe telling the truth. Metrics that track "speak-up" behaviors and the ability to raise concerns without retaliation reveal whether an institution is committed to learning or merely protecting itself.

A system committed to integrity would also track metrics of community health, like belonging and mutual respect. This would provide insight into whether teams were functioning as collections of individuals or as interdependent systems. When staff report feeling valued across roles and connected to one another, retention rates would almost certainly climb.

Lastly, integrity-focused healthcare systems track sustainability. They invest in recovery capital—emotional, relational, and institutional resources that allow people to rest, heal, and return after a crisis. Most importantly, they offer paid time off for healing. Metrics that measure access to support, the safety of stepping away (emotionally and financially), and the success of reintegration tell us whether a system is truly designed to support the people who maintain it.

In the end, integrity must apply to the entire institution, not just the individuals. If a department claims it values wellness, justice, transparency, or education, it should be able to show receipts. And it must ask hard questions: *Where do our incentives contradict our mission? Where are people punished for truth-telling? What behaviors are we rewarding in promotion, awards, and scheduling?* Integrity at the system level means the organization is willing to see itself clearly...and then change what it sees when necessary.

Systemic change in relation to integrity begins when we start measuring what really matters. Choosing metrics aligned with recovery sends a powerful message to those within the system: *you matter, your values matter, and your humanity is not collateral damage.* What we measure is what we become. If we want a healthcare system capable of healing others, it must first learn how to heal itself.

Final Thoughts

It's easy to feel overwhelmed by the dysfunction in healthcare. We often convince ourselves that nothing will change until the entire system does. And so we disengage. But the truth is that we don't need to fix the entire system to make a difference.

We rebuild integrity in the micro-moments of care and in the choices we make to show up differently. The moments may seem small, but they ripple outward. You don't have to change the system overnight. Just change the room you're in. And then the next one. And then the next. We recover healthcare with one moment of integrity at a time.

Reflection Questions

1. When was the last time you acted out of alignment with your values while at work? What contributed to that?
2. What are three core values that define the kind of provider and person you want to be?
3. In what ways do you justify small acts of misalignment? What are the costs of those justifications?
4. How can you begin to make space for integrity in micro-moments during a rushed shift, a difficult patient encounter, or a conflict with a colleague?

HOPE & UNCERTAINTY

The room was quiet in the way hospital rooms become quiet after something devastating has happened. The monitors were silenced. The mother, Lindsey, lay in bed staring at the ceiling, one hand resting on her abdomen, as if muscle memory had not yet caught up with reality. Her partner, the father, stood by the window, arms crossed tightly across his chest, staring out at the city lights below, willing himself not to fall apart. Lindsey came in for decreased fetal movement, and on evaluation, was diagnosed with an intrauterine fetal demise (IUFD).

The medical team did what medicine knows how to do. We explained the different etiologies of an IUFD. We answered questions about timelines, tests, and next steps. We offered choices where choices still existed. We spoke gently, clearly, and compassionately. And then, inevitably, we reached the edge of our language. The questions changed. *Why did this happen? What did we do wrong? How do we go on?* These are not questions that we are generally trained to answer in medicine. In the silence that followed, the weight of uncertainty pressed in on everyone in the room.

That was when the chaplain arrived.

He didn't come in with urgency or authority. He knocked softly, as if the room itself were fragile. Then he introduced himself and asked permission to sit. No agenda. Just presence. The chaplain pulled a chair close to the bed and waited. He allowed the grief to exist without interruption.

Lindsey was the first to speak, her voice barely audible. "I feel empty," she said. "I don't understand how my baby can be gone. We had a normal ultrasound just a few days ago."

The chaplain listened, eyes steady and posture open, not rushing her towards anything. When the father finally turned from the window with tears streaming down his face, the chaplain shifted slightly, widening the space so both of them could be held at once.

"I don't know how we're supposed to move forward," he said.

The chaplain didn't say that everything happens for a reason. He didn't try to explain the unexplainable. He simply acknowledged, "This is unbearable. And you don't have to carry it alone."

The chaplain followed up with gentle questions. What had they imagined for this child? Had they chosen a name? What did they want their baby to be remembered for? Slowly, stories emerged. A name was spoken aloud for the first time. A future that would never happen was named and grieved. The chaplain helped Lindsey and her partner create a small ritual, a moment to acknowledge that this life, though brief, mattered. That love had existed, and the loss was real.

No one suggested that another pregnancy would fix this. No one rushed them toward healing. Hope didn't arrive as optimism. In that room, hope had a quieter meaning. It meant being witnessed and held in the midst of devastation. It meant giving permission to grieve without having to understand. In that room, hope was simply the thing that helped this family take their next breath.

"You don't have to make sense of this today," the chaplain said. "You don't have to be strong. You don't have to know what comes next."

In a system that so often demands answers, the chaplain offered something radical: the reassurance that not knowing is okay. Medicine had carried this family to the edge of what could be explained. The chaplain had walked with them into what could not.

This is the kind of hope chaplains bring; it's the assurance that even when things are not okay, we're not alone. They teach us that healing doesn't always mean fixing and that uncertainty is an inevitable part of the healing process.

Medicine trains us to solve problems. We diagnose, explain, predict, and intervene. Certainty is often treated as competence. And yet, again and again, we run into moments that refuse to be explained. We face inconclusive tests, unpredictable outcomes, and suffering that arrives without warning. In those moments, the limits of medicine are laid bare.

What happens at that edge? When answers run out and uncertainty creeps in? That is where hope matters most, as a discipline of staying present in the unknown. Hope is less a feeling than a practice; it's the choice to remain connected when certainty fails.

Hope and Spirituality in Recovery

Two of the most essential principles in recovery are hope and spirituality. For me, the two are inseparable, for they both speak to my relationship with uncertainty. Both hope and spirituality require making the daily decision to keep going without guarantees, to loosen my grip on the illusion of control, and to trust that something beyond myself will meet me where I am.

That "something" does not need a specific name. It may be divine or communal, cosmic or quietly human. What matters is the belief that I don't have to carry everything alone. Hope and spirituality both recognize that support exists even when outcomes remain unclear.

The Second Step of Alcoholics Anonymous refers directly to these two principles. It reads, *"We came to believe that a Power greater than ourselves could restore us to sanity."* This step is often misunderstood or rejected, particularly by those who associate spirituality with institutional religion, coercion, or harm. That resistance is understandable. Many people have been wounded in the name of religion through exclusion, shame, or violence. The language of "God" or a "higher power" can feel more threatening than comforting.

What's often missed, however, is that the Twelve Steps are intentionally non-prescriptive. The phrase "a Power greater than ourselves" is deliberately open to interpretation. For some, it is Allah, Jesus, Krishna, or another deity. For others, it is the universe, nature, love, truth, or the collective wisdom of a recovery community. The point is not theology. The point is humility and the recognition that self-will alone is insufficient, and that healing requires a spiritual connection beyond the self.

I struggled with spirituality for a long time. Much of it felt confusing or inaccessible to me, especially as a gay boy who was raised Catholic in the Midwest. However, that began to shift after I watched the film *Conclave*, which centers on the election of a new pope. In one scene, a character reflects that faith is not born of certainty, but of uncertainty. He said that faith doesn't come from knowing. Rather, it comes from not knowing and believing anyway. That idea resonated deeply. I may not know what the future holds, but I can still believe that life is worth engaging, that healing is possible, and that I can continue forward even without answers. That's hope. That's spirituality. And both allow me to walk beside others as a companion in the mystery of healing.

In healthcare, however, spirituality is often neglected or dismissed altogether. It's treated as outside the scope of "real" medicine, as something sentimental or non-essential. The divide between science and religion is frequently framed as irreconcilable. In clinical settings, we leave little room for the unknown. We prioritize data, diagnoses, and deliverables while pushing mystery and the unknown to the margins. We chase certainty with the same desperation addicts chase a fix, believing that if we can know enough, control enough, and predict enough, we'll finally be competent providers.

The Cost of Certainty in Recovery

I know the seduction of certainty intimately. After my first experience in addiction treatment, I felt transformed in ways that were both real and intoxicating. My mind was clear again. The mental static that had once dominated my days was quiet. I woke up at the same time each morning. I went to work, exercised, and socialized with friends. For the first time in years, my life had structure, and structure felt like proof that I was fixed. I mistook early recovery momentum for permanence.

That sense of certainty felt like control. It gave me confidence. But I hadn't gained the quiet confidence of humility. It was the brittle confidence of finality. I began to believe I had it all figured out. I told myself I was different from others in recovery, that my insight, education, and self-awareness insulated me from relapse. I listened politely in peer-support meetings, but no longer felt I truly needed them. I started skipping days, then weeks. My sponsor's voice grew quieter in my life, replaced by my own internal narrative: *I'm fine now. I've learned my lesson. I'm certain I will remain sober.*

Certainty made me complacent. I stopped doing the daily work that had grounded me early on. I stopped checking in honestly about cravings, stress, or resentment. I stopped asking for help. I pulled away from the very community that had kept me alive. This behavior change didn't cause an immediate relapse. Instead, I drifted slowly and imperceptibly away from connection.

In hindsight, my relapse was inevitable. Certainty had closed me off from the practices that sustain recovery precisely because recovery is not a finish line. Over the years that followed, through multiple relapses and returns to treatment, I finally came to understand a truth that I now hold with reverence: addiction is a chronic, relapsing condition, and I do not know whether I will be sober forever. Not-knowing is what keeps me engaged.

Today, uncertainty is the cornerstone of my recovery, and it brings me back to meetings, back to my community, and back to honest conversations when life becomes overwhelming. It reminds me to pay attention to my internal state rather than assuming that I'm immune to old patterns. I no longer chase certainty. I take this one day at a time.

I don't know what tomorrow will bring. I don't know how future stressors will test me. But I know what is true today. Today, I am sober. Today, I am connected. Today, I am willing to ask for help. And today, I have hope. Not because I'm certain of the outcome, but because I am committed to the process.

The Cost of Certainty in Medicine

Certainty isn't healing, and more often than not, it's simply not possible. In medicine, certainty is often mistaken for competence, confidence, or strength. But when it becomes rigid, it carries serious unintended consequences. The drive for absolute answers can lead clinicians to over-diagnose, over-treat, or offer false reassurance in an attempt to appear in control.

This performance of certainty is often driven by fear rather than clinical necessity. It's the fear of appearing incompetent, of losing the trust of patients or colleagues. But when certainty becomes a performance, it undermines honesty, erodes patient autonomy, and reinforces a culture that treats vulnerability as weakness.

The consequences ripple outward. Patients may be led to believe there is only one "right" path forward, making it harder for them to cope when outcomes deviate from expectations. Clinicians, meanwhile, may feel isolated by the pressure to know everything. This results in shame, burnout, and moral injury when reality refuses to cooperate.

Perhaps most dangerously, certainty shuts down curiosity and connection. It silences second opinions, discourages collaboration, and prevents us from fully hearing the stories, values, and fears of the people we care for.

Hope, spirituality, and comfort with uncertainty are essential to whole-person care and to sustaining our humanity as clinicians. Despite extraordinary advances in diagnostics and therapeutics, uncertainty remains a constant in medicine. We cannot guarantee outcomes. We cannot predict every response. We cannot control illness, aging, or death.

Patients crave meaning, not just answers. They ask questions science alone cannot resolve: *Why is this happening? What does this mean for my life and my family? Will I be okay even if I am not cured?* Spirituality helps us make sense of our purpose, our identity, our grief, and our need to belong.

Hope provides emotional scaffolding, which allows us to hold onto the belief that something good is still possible even in suffering. Hope helps us keep showing up when a cure isn't' possible and reminds us that we aren't meant to carry the burden of responsibility alone. No clinician can cure everyone or fix every problem. That's too much for any one person to hold. Sometimes, hope means watching a patient leave despite your recommendations and trusting that the work will continue beyond you. And sometimes hope means accepting that a patient's journey may unfold in ways you did not choose and cannot control.

You're not to blame for what you cannot control. Control is an illusion. We exist within a vast, unpredictable universe. Medicine, at its best, is one person offering guidance, presence, and hope to another in this fragile, fleeting thing called life.

Into Practice

In my clinical work, I've had to redefine hope. I no longer think of hope as "hoping for a cure." I think of it as connection, comfort, and continuity. One of the simplest ways I practice this is by asking, "What are you hoping for today?" The answers are often not what I expect. Sometimes a patient hopes for pain control. Sometimes they hope to make it through the night. Sometimes they hope their partner will be engaged in conversations about their care. Sometimes they hope to feel less afraid. Naming those hopes gives us a shared direction.

When patients aren't sure what they're hoping for, I help them anchor goals of care in values. "What matters most to you right now? What are you most afraid of? What would a good day look like in this situation?"

I also offer hope without making promises I can't keep. I say things like, "I can't guarantee what will happen, but I can promise we will walk through this together." "We're going to make thoughtful decisions together, one step at a time." "There are still ways to bring comfort and meaning, even here." And I've learned to celebrate quiet victories for my patients. It might be a moment of rest, a decreased pain score, a family member arriving, another day pregnant, or just another deep breath.

One of the most powerful ways to build tolerance for uncertainty is to name it out loud. I sometimes say, "There are still things we don't know. That's hard. And we're going to stay with you while we figure out what we can." Naming uncertainty is honesty. And honesty builds trust.

Another way I practice uncertainty is to constantly question what I know. I am always looking things up, even guidelines that I've read dozens of times. I remain curious about advances in the field. Medicine moves so fast, and a healthy amount of uncertainty in my own knowledge helps me stay current with the latest literature. In other words, uncertainty helps me provide the best care possible.

In terms of spirituality, I strive to bring intentional acknowledgment to difficult cases. After a fetal loss or a traumatic delivery, I try and pause with the team before moving on. I refuse to let sacred moments be swallowed by the pace of medicine, and I invite spirituality in for both patients and colleagues alike. By honoring these moments, even briefly, I allow my teams to stay human within a system that often requires us to act more like machines.

Systemic Change

Healthcare systems are largely built to minimize uncertainty, yet much of clinical reality unfolds at the edge of what medicine can explain, predict, or fix. In those spaces, patients don't stop asking questions. The questions simply change. They become spiritual in nature: *Why is this happening? What does this mean for my life? Who am I now? How do I go on?*

Systems guided by hope and uncertainty recognize that these questions aren't peripheral to care. They are central. Designing healthcare that can truly meet patients where they are requires formally integrating spirituality into clinical care models across all types of illness, not just end-of-life care.

In practice, this begins with reframing spirituality as a universal human domain. Spirituality does not require belief in God, nor does it belong exclusively to chaplaincy or palliative care. It encompasses meaning, identity, values, connection, grief, and hope, dimensions present in every clinical encounter from prenatal care to oncology to primary care to addiction medicine. Systems aligned with hope acknowledge that addressing these dimensions is essential to whole-person healing. This means moving spiritual care out of the margins and embedding it into routine clinical workflows, patient assessments, and team-based models of care.

Clinicians cannot be expected to do this work without training. One of the most practical systems-level changes is the deliberate teaching of a shared language for what happens when medicine reaches its limits. We must teach clinicians how to sit with uncertainty, name it honestly, and offer hope without false reassurance. Learning this language should be treated as a core clinical skill, assessed and refined alongside physical exam techniques and procedural competence. Importantly, these competencies must be evaluated. Systems must integrate spiritual care and tolerance of uncertainty into assessments and professional expectations.

To support this, systems should require structured exposure to spiritual care through formal collaboration with chaplaincy services. Shadowing chaplains should be an expected part of clinical training, not an elective. Watching chaplains work teaches clinicians how to listen without fixing, hold silence, acknowledge grief without rushing it away, and help patients find meaning when answers are unavailable.

Additionally, patient intake forms and evaluations must include questions about spirituality, meaning, sources of strength, and what patients are hoping for. These questions invite the whole person into the clinical space by acknowledging that their inner lives matter.

Hope-centered systems also attend to the spiritual lives of clinicians themselves. Caring for patients at the edge of medicine requires internal resources that make space for spiritual practices among healthcare workers, whether that takes the form of mindfulness, meditation, prayer, reflective writing, or quiet time. When clinicians are permitted to tend to their own spirituality, they are better equipped to remain present with patients in moments of profound uncertainty.

When spirituality is integrated into clinical care models, we acknowledge that medicine operates within a larger human context that is defined by mystery, loss, and meaning. Systems that embrace hope and uncertainty do not abandon rigor; they deepen it. They allow clinicians and patients alike to remain truthful and engaged, even at the edge of what medicine can explain. And in doing so, they create the conditions for a quieter, more durable form of healing to take root.

Final Thoughts

Hope lives in the space between what we know and what we long for. Hope says, "*You are not alone. This moment still matters. There is still something worth holding onto.*" Hope and uncertainty are companions. Hope thrives in the unknown. It's not the absence of doubt. Rather, it's what arises in response to doubt. It is how we move forward, one uncertain step at a time, with faith that meaning, connection, and healing are still possible.

Reflection Questions

1. What role does spirituality play in how you understand suffering and healing?
2. Where in your work do you find it hardest to tolerate uncertainty? What practices help you remain grounded when outcomes are unclear?
3. What might it look like to integrate spiritual care more fully into your everyday practice?
4. When you encounter suffering that cannot be fixed, what does "good care" look like to you?

HUMILITY

I was always the first to arrive, the last to leave. The one who said yes to every teaching request, every extra shift, every administrative request. I became the go-to for everything. Precepting students. Covering for colleagues. Giving lectures. I wore my sacrifice like armor, and I seemed to run on a combination of caffeine, a constant need for recognition, and sometimes stimulants.

I wanted to be seen as dependable. I wanted to prove myself. I wanted to belong. But what I didn't realize at the time was that every "yes" I gave away at work was a quiet "no" to myself, my boundaries, and my recovery.

Somewhere along the way, my life outside of medicine quietly disappeared. My friendships thinned and hobbies faded. My apartment was a place to sleep, not to live. The phone never stopped buzzing, and I never stopped reaching for it. At one point, I hadn't taken a full day off in over a year because I was always available. And if you asked me why, I'd say, "Because they need me." But the truth was, I needed them, too. I needed to feel essential. Irreplaceable. Admired. My identity had collapsed into one word: Doctor.

The more I poured myself into work, the less attention I paid to my recovery.

Over the years, I've learned that recovery doesn't disappear all at once. It erodes slowly through missed meetings, skipped calls with my sponsor, and less socializing with friends. I told myself I was fine and that I could manage. But my addiction was patient. It waited in the shadows, doing push-ups, as they say.

Burnout crept in quietly, and by the time I realized how much of myself I had lost, there wasn't much left to give anyone, including myself. Every well-intentioned "yes" eventually caught up with me, and they brought me back to relapse. I wasn't saying yes out of service. I was saying yes out of fear and ego.

This chapter is for everyone who has confused being needed with being whole. Who has said yes out of fear, stayed late out of guilt, and slowly disappeared behind their identity in healthcare. The truth is, healing doesn't come from being everything to everyone. It comes from knowing you don't have to be.

The Threat of Ego

My habits of overfunctioning—staying late, avoiding delegation, never saying no—weren't just about work ethic. They were coping mechanisms and symptoms of a larger problem. For a long time, I confused overachieving with service. I believed that working harder, staying later, and doing more somehow made me a better doctor. Maybe even a better person. But that belief didn't come from a healthy sense of dedication. It came from ego and fear. I had a desperate need to prove that I was worthy of wearing my title of "doctor."

Some might wonder, *"How can being helpful to others be rooted in ego? Isn't that humility? Isn't it selflessness?"*

Not always. In fact, the most persistent forms of ego often disguise themselves as virtue.

I didn't fully grasp this until I came across the work of Eckhart Tolle. In *A New Earth*, he defines ego not as arrogance or bravado, but as a false sense of self that is built entirely on external identification, such as achievements, roles, opinions, credentials, thoughts, and status. In other words, the ego is the person we try to become in order to feel worthy.

I fully identified with my role as doctor. I was no longer Tony. I became Doctor Grandelis, entrusted with life and death, respected (or feared) in every room I walked into. It was intoxicating. And I very quickly forgot that medicine is my profession. Instead, medicine became who I was entirely.

Tolle explains that the ego thrives on comparison, control, and separation. It constantly seeks superiority, or sometimes inferiority, which can be just as self-centered. Ego draws its identity not from the present moment, but from the past (what I've achieved) and the future (what I fear or want). It attaches to thoughts and internal stories, mistaking them for truth.

My ego had me trapped in a never-ending narrative inside my head:

"I'm not doing enough."
"They can't handle this without me."
"If I stop working, I'll become irrelevant."
"If I don't answer, they'll be disappointed."
"If I don't perform, I'll be forgotten."

An acquaintance of mine once described the ego as the devil on your shoulder, telling you you're the best in the room one moment, and whispering you're a fraud the next. I've contended with both of those voices in my life. I've experienced the addictive highs of praise and accomplishment, and I've chased those feelings like a drug. I've also drowned in the lows of self-doubt, perfectionism, and people pleasing. That's ego, too.

In recovery, ego has often been my greatest barrier to healing. My ego has told me time and time again:

"You don't have a problem."
"You're not like those people."
"You're smarter than this. You can stop anytime."
And when I finally hit rock bottom, it morphed:
"You're broken."
"You're unlovable."
"No one could understand."
"You don't deserve help."

Ego kept me isolated, and it fed my shame. Recovery didn't truly begin until my ego cracked open, allowing space for humility to enter.

Ego in Medicine

Humility, in its truest form, is about knowing where you end and the rest of the world begins. In recovery, humility means admitting that we are powerless over our disease, that we need help, and that we are not in control.

In medicine, humility means acknowledging our limits, asking for support, sharing credit, and admitting when we don't know. It means understanding that our value isn't defined by how many patients we see, how many hours we work, or how well we perform. It's about being honest with ourselves and others.

But practicing humility is hard in a system that celebrates ego. Healthcare is often ruled by egoic behaviors. We've all met the surgeon who thinks they're untouchable or the intern who masks insecurity with bravado. There's the nurse who resents the team but refuses to speak up. And the attending who hasn't rested in weeks and wears exhaustion like a badge of honor.

Then there's the other kind of ego, the quieter, more insidious form, which says:

"If I'm not constantly needed, I have no value."
"If I set a boundary, they won't like me."
"If I say no, they'll think I'm lazy or selfish."

This is ego posing as martyrdom. And it's one of the most common causes of burnout in medicine today. We sacrifice ourselves to be the hero. When our worth becomes synonymous with our role, rest feels impossible. So, we over-function to feel secure and quietly grow resentful when no one sees how much we're holding. In the process, we forget that we're allowed to rest (that we must rest), and that asking for help or drawing a boundary is not weakness. It's integrity.

From Empathy to Ego

One patient encounter revealed how easy it was for me to slip from empathy into ego. The shift was subtle, almost imperceptible, but it changed the way I understood my role in the room.

A patient named Kathy came in late at night, guarded and exhausted, her body telling a story long before she put words to it. She'd been in a fight with her partner, and he had punched her in her pregnant abdomen. The chart listed a history of substance use, prior admissions for withdrawal, intermittent prenatal care, and a pattern of injuries explained away as accidents. When I walked into the room, Kathy met my eyes briefly and then looked away, as if deciding how much of herself it was safe to reveal.

As she talked, the pieces slowly came together. She was in active addiction. She had tried to stop at the beginning of pregnancy, but she relapsed. Her partner was unpredictable; sometimes apologetic, sometimes terrifying. She spoke in the language of self-blame, minimizing harm, and rationalizing her relationship with her partner. I recognized her fear instantly because I had lived inside it. I recognized the shame, the bargaining, the fragile hope that maybe things would be different this time.

I know the pull of substances as relief, as survival, as something that once felt like the only way to keep going. I also know what it's like to stay in relationships that harmed me, convinced that everything was fine or that brighter days were just around the corner. Sitting across from her, I felt an almost electric sense of identification. *I understand you*, I thought. *I've been here. I can help you.* And beneath that thought was something more dangerous: *I can save you...*

The rescuer instinct came online quickly and convincingly. I wanted to spend extra time in her room, to manage every detail of her care personally, to make exceptions, to smooth over conflicts, to ensure she never had to endure this trauma again. I imagined myself as the one doctor who would finally get it right. This is what ego looks like, disguised as empathy: I told myself that if I didn't do everything possible, I was failing her.

Humility required me to slow down and look honestly at what was happening inside me. My urge to fix was less about Kathy's needs and more about my identification with her suffering. I was blurring the boundary between connection and responsibility, between caring for someone and taking ownership of them.

As soon as I realized what was happening, I shifted course. Instead of promising what I couldn't deliver, I grounded myself in what ethical, sustainable care actually looks like. I acknowledged Kathy's fear without colluding with her self-blame. I spoke honestly about risks without using shame. I involved social work, addiction medicine, and advocates trained in intimate partner violence—people who, unlike myself, were professionally trained to manage these complex social factors. I made clear plans, named options, and reinforced that receiving help did not depend on perfection or compliance. Boundaries, in that moment, were not abandonment; they were respect for both of us.

Despite my attempts to detach from my rescuer role, I still carried Kathy with me when I left the hospital. That night, I replayed our conversation over and over again. I wondered if she would return to her partner. If she would use again. If I should have said something differently. This was the second edge of the lesson. I learned that my ego doesn't disappear when the shift ends; it follows me home, convincing me that either I did something wrong, didn't do enough, or, conversely, am the only one who can truly help.

That encounter forced me to confront an essential truth: My history allows me to connect deeply with patients, but it does not give me ownership over their outcomes. Shared pain can build trust, but it can also erode boundaries. Humility lives in knowing where I end and another person begins. Healing isn't something I can impose or will into existence. Sometimes the most honest act of care is to show up fully, offer what is mine to offer, and then step back. This requires me to trust that change, like recovery, happens in its own time—and never because one person decided to carry it all.

Into Practice

In both recovery and healthcare, I've learned that "no" is not rejection or failure. It's an act of spiritual maturity. It's a declaration of self-awareness, healthy boundaries, and trust in others. It is one of the simplest ways I can honor my integrity.

Whereas saying "no" used to feel like selfishness to me, now I see it as the powerful recognition that I am not limitless. I am not indispensable. I am not the solution to every problem. And I'm not supposed to be. This kind of humility helps me discern what is mine to carry and what is not. It creates space for others to step in, step up, and shine.

When I say no with clarity and compassion, I'm drawing a boundary that protects my time as well as my spirit. In recovery, boundaries are lifesaving. I've learned to say no to people, places, and things that destabilize me. In healthcare, I've learned to use these same boundaries:

"No, I can't pick up another shift."
"No, I'm not available after hours."
"No, I'm unable to respond to messages on my day off."

Saying no doesn't have to be harsh or defensive. In fact, it can be kind and connective. Here are some gentle, grounding ways I practice it:

"I trust you to handle this."
"I'm not able to take this on right now."
"This isn't aligned with my values or capacity."
"I need to honor my limits, and that means saying no to this."
"Let's revisit this when I have more space."

Humility, for me, is practiced most honestly through boundaries, through learning when to step back rather than step in. This is a daily spiritual discipline that requires self-awareness, restraint, and trust. Before responding to requests or opportunities, I intentionally pause and check in with myself. I ask whether I'm acting from ego, fear, or genuine service. I notice when my sense of worth becomes entangled with being needed, when guilt masquerades as generosity, or when over-functioning feels easier than tolerating uncertainty. These moments of reflection help me move from impulse to intention and remind me that not every problem requires my intervention.

I also practice humility by acknowledging that stepping back doesn't mean abandoning responsibility. I reflect on moments when I chose not to fix things and then noticed something meaningful emerge anyway. Times when asking for help strengthened my relationships rather than weakened them.

Times when saying no created space for others to grow or for my own energy to be restored. Holding these memories counters the belief that everything depends on me and reinforces the deeper truth that the world continues, and often improves, when I relinquish control.

Maintaining boundaries requires intentional pacing. When asked to take on additional responsibilities, especially in real-time and face-to-face, I give myself permission to pause. I no longer feel compelled to decide immediately. Instead, I say, "Let me think about this and get back to you," creating space to respond thoughtfully rather than reactively. I often choose to follow up by email or text, knowing that clarity and honesty are easier when urgency is removed. This practice respects my limits, my values, and the quality of the commitments I choose to make.

Systemic Change

Systems guided by humility are built on the recognition that no individual is limitless, indispensable, or meant to carry the weight of care alone. In healthcare, this requires designing structures that protect those limits rather than exploit them. A humble system doesn't reward self-sacrifice masquerading as dedication. Nor does it depend on a few overfunctioning individuals to compensate for structural deficiencies. Instead, it distributes responsibilities, enforces rest, and treats sustainability as a core patient-safety principle.

One of the most concrete expressions of humility at the systems level is how time off is tracked and protected. In a humility-guided system, time off is tracked as a safety metric. Leaders monitor not only hours worked, but days off, recovery time after overnight or 24-hour shifts, and patterns of chronic overextension.

When clinicians go long stretches without rest, this is treated as a warning signal, not a badge of honor. Mandatory recovery periods after extended shifts, protected post-call time, and enforced limits on consecutive workdays reflect an institutional acknowledgment of biological reality. Exhausted clinicians are not safer, wiser, or more virtuous. To the contrary, they're more vulnerable, error-prone, and at risk of harm to themselves and others.

Humility also requires formal limits on the accumulation of responsibility. A humility-based model requires explicit review before additional responsibilities are assigned. Teaching requests, leadership roles, committee work, extra shifts, and administrative tasks are evaluated in the context of a clinician's existing load. No one is allowed to take on more without a clear accounting of what they are already holding.

Equally important are structural protections around communication. Systems that expect constant availability (such as instant replies to emails, texts, pages, or messages) create a profound boundary violation that feeds the ego. The implicit message is: *your worth is tied to your responsiveness.* Humility-guided systems dismantle this expectation. They establish clear norms for response times, protect off-hours from non-urgent communication, and model delayed responses from leadership. When immediacy is no longer the default, clinicians are freed from the illusion that they must always be "on" to be valued.

Training in humility must also be taught and reinforced. Clinicians need explicit education in boundary-setting as a clinical skill. Learning to say no clearly, to pause before committing, and to tolerate guilt without collapsing into compliance are essential competencies for sustainable practice. Systems grounded in humility normalize phrases like, "Let me review my capacity," "I'm not able to take this on right now," and "This needs to be a shared responsibility."

Healthcare doesn't need more heroes. It needs structures that make heroism unnecessary. A humility-based system recognizes that healing relies on knowing our limits, honoring them collectively, and trusting that care can continue even when we step back.

Final Thoughts

Humility doesn't ask us to shrink or disengage; it asks us to recognize what is truly ours to carry. From this standpoint, boundaries are acts of clarity. They help us be clear about our limits, our values, and the role we're meant to play in any given moment. When ego drives us, we overextend and over-function. We confuse indispensability with worth. When humility leads, we learn to step back without abandoning care.

In recovery and in medicine alike, boundaries protect integrity. They allow us to stay present rather than depleted. Boundaries allow generosity to remain genuine, unburdened by the resentment that grows when we give beyond our capacity. In short, learning to serve without losing ourselves is how we stay in this work with honesty, sustainability, and grace.

Reflection Questions

1. When have you said yes out of fear, guilt, or the need to feel important?
2. In what ways do you confuse your professional identity with your personal worth?

3. What messages have you received that make saying no difficult for you?
4. Who in your life models humility well? What can you learn from them?
5. What professional boundaries do you need to revisit? Which ones do you need to create for the first time?

AUTHENTICITY & CURIOSITY

I was two years into my first job as an attending physician. I had worked on Labor & Delivery long enough to know the rhythm of the floor—when to lean in and when to let go, when to lead and when to step back. It was the start of a new academic year, and the upcoming second-year residents were in charge of running the labor floor. Alicia was the first resident to rotate through that year.

At first, I thought Alicia might just be having a bad day. During morning rounds, I gently suggested a different way she could have managed a non-reassuring fetal heart rate tracing overnight. She stiffened. "I just did what I was told to do last week," she said, tight-lipped.

I nodded, letting it go for the moment. But over the next few days, a pattern emerged. Each time I offered guidance on routine matters like documentation, counseling techniques, or surgical efficiency, Alicia met me with a wall of resistance.

"I'm doing exactly what you taught me."

"The patient didn't seem to mind."

"Well, that's not what Dr. X said last time."

Her posture was guarded, and her tone was generally polite but clipped.

Alicia didn't realize it, but she wasn't learning because she was spending more energy defending herself rather than reflecting. The team started to feel it, too. Nurses hesitated to bring up concerns. Her junior residents stopped asking questions. I stopped giving feedback.

One night, after a tense shoulder dystocia, I debriefed with her. I tried to praise what she did well while suggesting ways to prepare for future emergencies. She immediately interrupted, "I got the baby out in under two minutes. I'd say that's pretty good. We can't be expected to be perfect yet."

"No one is asking you to be perfect," I said gently. "But are you open to feedback?"

She stared at me and then looked away.

In that moment, I realized two things. 1) Unsolicited advice is never the right approach. 2) Responding defensively effectively shuts off the opportunity for continued growth and learning.

Over the next few weeks, I took a different approach. I praised Alicia's clinical wins and invited her to reflect before giving feedback. I asked questions instead of giving directives. "What felt hard about that delivery?" What would you do differently next time?" Gradually, Alicia started to soften.

One evening, after a particularly long day, Alicia stayed behind to finish notes. On her way out, she found me at a computer in the workroom. "Dr. Grandelis," she said quietly. "I've been thinking about what you said....about being open. I guess I've been afraid that if I admit I don't know something or make a mistake, people will think I'm a bad doctor."

I looked up. "Alicia, the strongest physicians I know are the ones who ask for help."

She nodded, her eyes gazing at the floor. "I'm trying."

Over the following months, Alicia's posture changed. She had less armor, more curiosity. She started soliciting feedback before it was offered. Her patient care improved because she reflected rather than defended. Patients sensed her calm, nurses trusted her again, and interns sought her out to learn from her. By the end of the year, Alicia was becoming the kind of physician others looked up to. And it all started with a conversation she almost didn't let herself hear.

DEFENSIVENESS

One of the most important lessons I try to teach new interns has nothing to do with medicine and everything to do with awareness. Notice when you're being defensive. Notice it in the tone of your voice, the quickness of your reply, and the impulse to explain, justify, or shift the blame. When you feel that heat rising—pause. That momentary pause can change everything.

I teach this not because I've mastered it, but because it's one of my greatest character flaws. I was Alicia, the resident who couldn't hear feedback without bristling. In some ways, I still am. The difference today is that I can see it coming. I can feel that instinct to defend myself from perceived attack. And I'm learning, with time and humility, how to shift before it overtakes me.

Defensiveness wasn't something that only showed up in my clinical training. It showed up everywhere. It surfaced in conversations with friends, in faculty meetings, and especially in romantic relationships. If someone pointed out a way I'd hurt them or something I could improve, I'd leap to defend myself. Oftentimes, I'd turn it back on them, countering, "Well, what about you?"

Inadequacy and Shame

It wasn't until I got sober that I began to untangle the roots of my defensiveness. And what I found at the core of it all was a deep, pervasive sense of inadequacy.

That feeling started early in life. I'd been surrounded by unspoken rules about what boys were supposed to be, rules I forced myself to follow. I wanted desperately not to be gay. When I realized I couldn't change that about myself, I internalized a belief that there was something wrong with me. That I was broken. That I didn't belong.

That sense of not belonging followed me into college, then into medical school, and finally into residency. Residency, in particular, was brutal. I felt like an imposter every day, constantly questioning whether I was smart enough to be a doctor. As one of few men in a medical specialty dominated by women, I convinced myself that patients didn't want to see me. I was certain they were disappointed when I walked into the room because I was a male.

So, you can imagine how I reacted when I received feedback that challenged my clinical judgment or competence. I would shut it down immediately. Externally, I reacted with explanation, but internally, I withered with shame. Because to admit even a small mistake felt like opening the floodgates to a lifelong fear: *Maybe they're right. Maybe I don't belong here. Maybe I never did.*

When that fear got too loud, too unbearable, the only way I knew how to quiet it was with substances. Drugs and alcohol were my armor against inadequacy.

I've come to understand that defensiveness is a shield I use to protect myself from shame. It's how I cope with the fear of inadequacy. That fear is not unique to me or people with substance use disorders. It's part of the human condition.

In medicine, I've been trained to hide my insecurities. I always felt like I was expected to be competent and unshakeable. There never seemed to be room for doubt, or the messy, human parts of growth. So I hid behind a mask of confidence. When I received feedback, I told myself I was being misunderstood or that the criticism was unfair. But really, I was protecting myself from feeling like a failure.

Those who struggle the most with feedback are often the ones who care the most. We're the ones who desperately want to be good and to prove our worth. But instead of owning that vulnerability, we armor ourselves with defensiveness. In doing so, we rob ourselves of the very thing we need most: growth.

The Power of Honest Reflection

Step 4 in the Twelve Steps of recovery asked me to "make a searching and fearless moral inventory of myself."

As I see it, this step is about honest reflection. It requires willingness to see myself fully, to name my character defects, and to understand the patterns I use to protect my ego. Step 4, in many ways, mirrors what I ask trainees to do when they receive feedback. Look within. Reflect. Ask yourself, "Is there something here I can grow from?"

When a trainee becomes defensive, the openness to change closes. Defensiveness builds a wall that pushes away supervisors and blocks opportunities for mentorship, which limits learning. And in a profession that relies on lifelong learning, that's a dangerous place to stay.

We don't grow by being perfect. We grow by staying willing. Willing to listen. Willing to learn. Willing to sit with discomfort. Willing to admit when we're wrong. Willing to stay curious. Willing to stay authentic to our true selves.

The truth is, we will all make mistakes. We will all fall short. But our worth isn't determined by how few mistakes we make. It's determined by how we respond to them.

Into Practice

Recovery has taught me that I don't always have to get it right. I just have to remain curious about myself and accept who I am and where I am on this journey. The same is true in medicine. When I stop struggling for perfection and start striving for openness and integrity, the path forward becomes lighter. The work becomes less lonely, and it becomes crystal clear to me that I do belong. Reflecting honestly on myself helps me to show up in my true, authentic form.

This transformation has taken time, though, and the first step has been noticing when I become defensive. Defensiveness can take many forms for me, including sarcasm, silence, over-explaining, blame, and withdrawal. But by learning to recognize these responses, I can stop them from materializing and, in turn, leave myself open to authentic curiosity and personal growth.

Below is a list of common defensive responses that I've noticed in myself and others over the years. Start to identify and acknowledge if you use any of these phrases. Awareness is the first step toward change.

Denial & Dismissal

"I know."

"I don't think that actually happened."

"That's not what I was trying to do."

"I've never had an issue with that before."

"I don't think that's really a problem."

Rationalization & Justification

"I was just following what I saw someone else do."

"I had a lot on my plate that day."

"The patient was really difficult to work with."

"I didn't have enough time."

Blaming External Factors

"I wasn't given clear instructions."

"The attending didn't explain it well."

"The nurses didn't tell me what was going on."

"The patient was non-compliant, so there was nothing I could do."

Minimization

"It really doesn't seem like that big of a deal."

"Other people do the same thing."

"I don't usually do it like that."

"That's just my style of doing things."

Shifting the Focus

"But I did everything else right!"

"What about all the things I did well?"

"Other people did the same thing, why am I the only one getting feedback?"

Emotional Reactions

"This feels really unfair."

"I don't think you understand how hard I've been working."

"This is making me feel like I'm not good enough."

"I don't even know why I'm being criticized for this."

Avoidance & Deflection

"I get it. Can we move on?"

"Noted." (when said dismissively)

Overgeneralization & Catastrophizing

"I can't seem to do anything right."

"Maybe I'm not cut out for this."

"No matter what I do, I just get criticized."

SYSTEMIC CHANGE

Systems guided by authenticity and curiosity would intentionally be designed to make learning safer. They would create environments that support clinicians in asking questions and reflecting honestly on their work.

This begins with a fundamental shift in how feedback is structured and delivered. Rather than relying on unsolicited correction, anonymous written evaluations, or top-down critique, curiosity-driven systems normalize reflective dialogue. Feedback is preceded by invitation and grounded in shared goals. It's framed as an opportunity for growth, with questions like, "What felt challenging about that?" and "What would you want to try differently next time?" These kinds of questions would be embedded into routine clinical interactions and debrief checklists.

Feedback needs to work both ways as well. Trainees aren't the only ones who need feedback. Our leaders need to be open and receptive as well. This means offering frequent opportunities to give feedback to departmental leadership and instructing attending physicians on how to elicit feedback for themselves.

Authenticity at the systems level also requires dismantling the culture of shame that fuels defensiveness. Evaluation frameworks must distinguish between mistakes and identity. When clinicians and trainees fear that admitting uncertainty or error will label them as incompetent, they predictably protect themselves by rationalizing, minimizing, or deflecting. Curiosity and growth cannot survive in that environment.

Systems aligned with authenticity also reward reflective capacity, such as the ability to name mistakes, integrate feedback, and demonstrate growth over time. Assessments would track not only outcomes but openness, examining whether clinicians solicit feedback, how they respond to it, and whether they can articulate lessons learned.

Training programs must also teach awareness of defensiveness as a universal human response. Medical education should help clinicians recognize the early signals of defensiveness (tightening posture, rapid justification, emotional heat) and pause before reacting. Teaching clinicians to notice their internal reactions and remain curious would directly improve learning, collaboration with colleagues, and patient safety.

Finally, systems can make curiosity practical by giving it a home in the schedule. What if we held a different type of M&M conference? What if instead of "Morbidity & Mortality," we had "Meaning & Moments" conferences where the focus is on curiosity, asking questions such as:

"What made this case meaningful for the team involved?"
"What moment changed the trajectory of this case?"
"What emotions came up during this case?
"How did these emotions influence clinical decision making?"
"Where could assumptions or biases have shown up?"
"Could more space have been made for vulnerability?"
"What can we take away from this case as clinicians?
'What can we take away from this case as humans?"
"Would we approach this case differently in the future?"

"What did we learn about the kind of providers we want to be?"

"What would you want a trainee to learn from this case?"

"Could we have slowed down? Would the outcome differ?"

"How did we communicate uncertainty, risk, or bad news?"

"Did the patient feel seen and heard throughout their care?"

"Were there constraints that shaped our decisions in ways we may not have noticed at the time?"

Final Thoughts

This chapter is a call to return to our most authentic selves. When we move beyond defensiveness and perfectionism, we can finally stop trying to prove our worth and start discovering who we are beneath the armor.

If we can meet our fear, shame, and even our missteps with that kind of wondering, it unlocks a new path forward. We don't have to have all the answers, only the courage to ask the right questions.

REFLECTION QUESTIONS

1. When was the last time you noticed yourself becoming defensive at work? What was underneath your reaction?
2. What does curiosity look like for you in your day-to-day practice?
3. Are there certain people or situations that make it harder for you to receive feedback openly? Why do you think that is?
4. What does authentic leadership mean to you? How do you model that for others?

FORGIVENESS

In recovery, we learn that forgiveness is not a one-time act. It's a process. That process is sometimes slow and painful, but it is always essential. We forgive others because we deserve peace, and we forgive ourselves because self-forgiveness is about recognizing that we are more than what we've done.

In medicine, however, forgiveness is rarely discussed. Our training emphasizes precision, accountability, and performance. We're taught to chart every detail, anticipate every risk, and never, ever make a mistake. And if we do make one? The unspoken message is: Don't let it happen again.

There's little room for grace in a culture built on perfectionism. But no matter how careful we are, we will all get it wrong sometimes. And without forgiveness—real, compassionate, honest forgiveness—we carry those mistakes like lead in our chest.

The Weight of Self-Blame

I once carried enormous shame about my addiction. Even after entering recovery, I couldn't forgive myself for the person I had become during the worst of it. I was unreliable, emotionally absent, and consumed by secrecy. I replayed the moments when I hurt loved ones or let colleagues down. I thought about the times I avoided my friends or hid behind a smile that masked the chaos.

When I first started telling my story publicly, I did so with caution. I framed it in ways that would make others more comfortable. I softened the edges. But no matter how I told it, I still felt a residue of guilt afterward. Because some part of me still believed: *if you had just been stronger, smarter, more disciplined, none of this would have happened.*

It wasn't until I heard my sponsor share his story, with honesty and humility, that I felt a change take root in me. He didn't sugarcoat. He didn't minimize. He just owned it. That night, I did something I hadn't done since getting sober. I forgave myself. I said it aloud. And I meant it.

Once I was able to forgive myself, I began asking others for forgiveness. In recovery circles, Steps 8 and 9 ask us to make a list of people whom we have harmed as a direct result of our drug or alcohol use. Then, we are invited to make amends to such people. This process has been slow and uncomfortable for me. But what I've learned is that making amends isn't about earning absolution or asking someone else to relieve us of our guilt; it's about taking responsibility without defensiveness, conditions, or expectations.

In recovery, an amend is an act of integrity. It says: *I see clearly now what my actions did. I am not asking you to make me feel better. I am here to name the harm, to own it, and to change my behavior going forward.* That shift—from seeking forgiveness to practicing accountability—moved me out of self-centered shame and into relational honesty.

What surprised me most is that amends are as much about forgiving myself as they are about repairing relationships. Some amends I've made have been welcomed; others have been met with silence, anger, or a door that stays firmly closed. Recovery has taught me that I do not control the outcome, only the sincerity of the effort. I've also learned that sometimes an amend is not an apology at all. Instead, it's changed conduct. This is called a "living amends," and over time, these amends become a daily practice. It's a commitment to align our values with our actions. Forgiveness, then, isn't about forgetting the past. It's about refusing to let it dictate who we become next.

Forgiveness in Healthcare

There was a moment early in my attending career when I unintentionally asked a resident to act against her values. We were on call together, and the unit was full. A patient with an uncomplicated pregnancy had presented in early labor. The resident, Lauren, was assigned to her.

After a long night, the patient delivered, but the placenta wouldn't come. Lauren called me in, exhausted, and I told her to remove it manually. The patient cried out in pain, and Lauren froze. "She doesn't have adequate analgesia," she whispered.

I was tired. I just wanted the case done. I told her to proceed and informed the patient that it would be over and done quickly.

If she were in pain, she could squeeze the nurse's hand. Lauren hesitated, then did as she was told. We managed the placenta, the bleeding stopped, and the patient remained stable. But after we left the room, Lauren looked stricken.

Later that day, she found me in the workroom. "I need to say something," she said. Her voice was steady but low. "I don't feel great about that delivery. I don't think that was right, to proceed without adequate pain control."

I was caught off guard. But in that moment, I remembered what it felt like to go against your gut and then carry that feeling with you for days, weeks, years. I remembered what it felt like to not speak up.

I looked at her and said, "You're right. I was wrong to ask you to do that. And I'm sorry. I will apologize to the patient, too."

Lauren nodded. "Thank you," she said.

I think about that moment often. Not because it was a huge clinical error. It wasn't. But because it was a moment where someone trusted me with their moral compass, and I veered it off course.

That day taught me that one of the greatest responsibilities of leadership is to listen when someone tells you they've been hurt. My role is not to defend or justify, but to simply say: "I hear you. I'm sorry. What can I do to make it right?"

Forgiveness in healthcare is a radical act. It pushes against the grain of our perfectionist, punitive culture. It invites nuance into a world that too often sees in black-and-white. And it allows us to keep going together.

We need to forgive our colleagues when they fall short. We need to forgive trainees for not knowing yet. We need to forgive leaders who are learning as they go. And most of all, we need to forgive ourselves because we cannot be both judge and healer at once.

Forgiveness is not forgetting. It's about remembering with compassion as we gently hold people accountable (including ourselves). It's choosing to believe that who someone is becoming matters more than who they were at their worst.

And we must also learn that forgiveness isn't always something we need to seek. The number of times I hear "I'm sorry" from trainees is staggering. They apologize for asking questions, for not knowing something, for being unsure, or for forgetting to order a lab or obtain a pertinent piece of a patient's history. They are essentially apologizing for existing in a space where learning is supposed to happen. Why? Because the system has conditioned them to believe they must be perfect, that anything less is failure.

Yes, there are moments when an apology is appropriate. But more often, I gently interrupt: "You have nothing to apologize for. That was not a mistake. That was learning."

Growth should never make us feel ashamed.

More On Apologies

In her book, *Why Won't You Apologize? Healing Big Betrayals and Everyday Hurts*, psychologist Harriet Lerner explores the psychology of apologies; what makes them meaningful, why we avoid giving them, and how to cope when we never receive one. Dr. Lerner emphasizes that a true apology is not about defending oneself or minimizing harm. It's about taking full responsibility for the impact of one's actions without justification, blame-shifting, or performance.

She identifies the most common barriers to apology, such as shame, perfectionism, and fear of losing power or moral high ground. These are all themes that resonate deeply in medical culture, where trainees and attendings alike may struggle to admit mistakes due to fear of judgment, litigation, or institutional repercussions.

One of Lerner's most powerful teachings is that an apology is not about erasing what happened. Rather, it's about validating the other person's experience and demonstrating a willingness to repair the relationship.

Dr. Lerner's insights are especially relevant for people in the medical profession. The overuse of apologies among medical trainees isn't always about genuine remorse. Instead, it's often a symptom of internalized shame combined with the unrealistic standards set by our training systems. At the same time, the lack of meaningful apologies from those in power—especially after public humiliation, harsh criticism, or institutional failures—reinforces a culture of silence and fear.

By learning what a genuine apology looks like, and when it's actually needed, we can foster a culture that values authentic accountability over performative guilt, and self-compassion over perfectionism. We can also begin to forgive ourselves and each other, not because we're excusing harm, but because we're choosing to move forward with honesty and grace.

Into Practice

For much of my training and early career in healthcare, apology felt incompatible with authority. In clinical spaces shaped by hierarchy, evaluations, and legal fear, apology felt risky. I worried that acknowledging harm would undermine my credibility with learners, weaken my leadership, or expose me professionally. What recovery has taught me, and what medical education rarely names explicitly, is that apology is not a failure of authority. It's one of the most ethical expressions an authority figure can make. This understanding, along with Harriet Lerner's teachings, has completely revolutionized how I practice giving and receiving apologies, as well as how I understand forgiveness.

Learning how to apologize as a clinician required me to confront how often my words and actions carried more weight than I intended. A comment made during rounds, a teaching point delivered too sharply, or a clinical decision made quickly under pressure can land with disproportionate impact on others. I've learned that a meaningful apology in these settings must be specific and direct. Instead of defaulting to vague language like "Sorry if that came off wrong," I practice naming the behavior and its impact: "When I corrected you in front of the team during rounds, I embarrassed you. That wasn't fair, and I'm sorry." This kind of clarity strengthens trust and models accountability in real time.

One of the hardest habits for me to break was explaining myself when apologizing. In medicine, we're trained to contextualize everything. But I've learned that when I'm apologizing to a trainee or colleague, explanations often function as defenses. Saying "I was under a lot of pressure" or "That's how I was trained" may be true, but it shifts the focus away from impact. As an educator, I now try to pause, own my part without qualification, and resist the urge to make myself feel better in the moment.

Receiving apologies within the healthcare hierarchy has been just as instructive. When a supervisor, colleague, or learner apologizes to me, I've noticed how tempting it can be to dismiss the moment quickly, especially when power dynamics are involved. Early on, I often said, "It's fine," even when it wasn't, partly to keep things moving and partly to avoid discomfort.

However, what I've learned is that minimizing harm helps no one, and it can prevent both parties from healing. Now, when someone apologizes, I try to slow the moment down. I acknowledge the courage it takes to say the words out loud, and I'm honest about the impact: "Thank you for saying that. That interaction we had in front of the patient earlier really stayed with me." Accepting an apology without erasing the experience has allowed for deeper trust and more authentic professional relationships.

When I practice apology, receive it with presence, and ask for forgiveness when appropriate, I create a learning environment grounded in trust rather than fear. These practices remind me that practicing medicine is about being accountable, reflective, and willing to repair. In a profession that often rewards silence and self-protection, choosing to apologize and forgive has become one of the most meaningful ways I practice integrity.

Systemic Change

Systemic change around forgiveness in medicine begins by moving away from a culture that treats mistakes as personal failures and towards one that understands misjudgment and growth as inevitable parts of human work. Practically, this means redesigning how institutions respond when things go wrong. As mentioned in previous chapters, peer review committees, for example, can shift from thinly veiled blame sessions to true learning and repair spaces where the first question is not "Who messed up?" but "What happened, what was the impact, and what support is needed for everyone involved?" Including a brief, explicit acknowledgment of emotional and moral impact on clinicians (not just clinical outcomes) signals that forgiveness and repair are part of professional practice, not signs of weakness.

Another concrete change is separating accountability from punishment. Many clinicians resist honesty and apology because they fear formal repercussions, including negative evaluations, lost opportunities, or legal exposure. Systems can counter this by creating protected pathways for disclosure, apology, and repair, similar to peer support or second-victim programs. For instance, when a clinician makes a mistake or harms a colleague, there could be a structured, confidential process facilitated by trained peers or mediators that focuses on understanding the impact, offering an apology, and identifying repair opportunities. When people trust that telling the truth won't have major professional consequences, forgiveness becomes possible.

Training environments, in particular, need to normalize learning without shame. One practical intervention is to explicitly coach trainees on when apologies are appropriate and when they are not. Program leadership can say out loud, repeatedly, "You do not need to apologize for learning." Attendings can model this by gently interrupting reflexive apologies and reframing them: "You didn't do anything wrong; this is part of training," or "Thank you for asking; that's exactly what you're supposed to do." Over time, this helps dismantle the internalized belief that imperfection requires self-punishment and opens space for self-forgiveness.

Leadership behavior is, perhaps, the most powerful lever for systemic change. When leaders never apologize, forgiveness becomes aspirational rather than real. But when a department chair, medical director, or attending publicly says, "I handled that poorly," or "I'm sorry for the impact that decision had on the team," it resets what is permissible. Practical examples include leaders apologizing after harsh emails, owning miscommunications in staff meetings, or acknowledging when policies caused unintended harm. These moments don't undermine authority. Rather, they humanize it and teach that repair is part of professionalism.

In this kind of system, forgiveness is no longer something individuals have to fight for on their own. It's woven into how teams learn, how leaders lead, and how institutions respond to harm. In that type of environment, people can make mistakes and tell the truth about them. Then, they can focus on repairing any damage and move forward. They won't be defined by their worst moment, but shaped by how they grew from it.

Final Thoughts

Forgiveness is a practice. And like any practice, it takes repetition, attention, and intention. Some days you will do it well. Other days, the old narratives will pull you back. But keep practicing. Say the words out loud. Send the text. Call the person. Let the apology be awkward. Let it be messy. Over time, forgiveness will take root. And from that root, something stronger will grow.

Reflection Questions

1. What is something from your past that you struggle to forgive yourself for? What would it look like to begin letting go?
2. Have you ever asked someone for forgiveness in a professional setting? What held you back or helped you move forward?
3. When was the last time you received a meaningful apology? What made it feel genuine or healing?
4. Do you find yourself over-apologizing at work? Why do you think you do that?
5. If someone came to you today asking for forgiveness, how would you want to respond?

A WORD ABOUT RESILIENCE

The longer I've practiced medicine, the more increasingly uncomfortable I've grown with the word *resilience.* It's meant to inspire. But over time, it has grown heavier and heavier, particularly as it's used in healthcare and medical training.

We hold resilience up like a virtue in medicine. We praise people for their toughness, for pushing through pain. But in the world of addiction, resilience is often the very thing that kills us. By definition, resilience means the capacity to withstand or recover quickly from difficulties. It implies grit. Endurance. Fortitude. But for those of us with substance use disorders, that kind of toughness becomes dangerous. We do withstand a lot. We do push through. We keep showing up, long after we've stopped coping. We survive metaphorical fires that are burning our lives to the ground.

Until we don't.

Until we overdose.

Until we die.

So, you can imagine why resilience doesn't sit well with me.

In recovery, I've learned that healing doesn't come from white-knuckling your way through life. It comes from surrender and softness. It comes from asking for help when you're not okay. That is the strength that saves us.

So, when I hear resilience used as a benchmark for how "well" someone is doing, especially in medicine, I flinch. Not because I think resilience is bad. But because I know it's incomplete. *Sometimes, the bravest thing a person can do is not be resilient at all.* We all have moments when we need to stop and rest. Sometimes we even need to fall apart and let someone else help hold the pieces.

The Danger of Resilience in Healthcare

In healthcare, resilience has become a buzzword for strength and perseverance. We're told to "be resilient" through long shifts and traumatic cases. It's stitched into wellness workshops, ever-present in evaluation feedback, and embedded in institutional values. But beneath its well-meaning surface, resilience can be a dangerously loaded expectation.

The problem isn't resilience itself. It's the demand for it. When resilience becomes the metric by which healthcare professionals are judged or a benchmark for how "well" someone is doing, it morphs from an internal strength to an external pressure. It tells us that when the system fails, when support is absent, when trauma accumulates, and when we reach our emotional limits, the solution is to push through. Try harder. Don't complain.

This framing shifts the burden of coping away from the system and onto the individual. It implies that if you're struggling, it's a personal failure of toughness, not a natural response to dehumanizing conditions. This attitude perpetuates the stigma around mental health by creating a culture where vulnerability is punished, not protected.

The truth is, we cannot always be resilient, nor should we be expected to. Sometimes, we're exhausted. Sometimes, we're overwhelmed by grief or trauma. Sometimes, what we need is not to "bounce back," but to stop and rest. The work of healing requires more than stamina. It requires space, safety, and compassion.

If we want to create a sustainable future in healthcare, we must stop worshipping resilience and start building systems that don't require it as a survival strategy. We must validate the moments when resilience isn't possible. And we must redefine strength, not as stoicism in the face of suffering, but as the courage to say, "I need help."

Final Thoughts

Resilience has a place in medicine, but it cannot be the place where we end the conversation. When resilience becomes the answer to suffering rather than a response to being supported, it quietly excuses broken systems. It silences those who are struggling most. Recovery taught me that real strength is not endless endurance; it's discernment—knowing when to keep going and when to stop, ask for help, and let yourself be held. If healthcare is ever going to heal, we must create environments where people are not admired for surviving harm, but protected from it in the first place. A sustainable, humane system does not require its workforce to be resilient just to stay alive within it.

Reflection Questions

1. When have you been praised for being "resilient" when what you actually needed was support?
2. In your training or workplace, how is resilience rewarded, and what vulnerabilities are quietly discouraged?
3. How do your institution's policies place the burden of coping on individuals instead of addressing systemic harm?

THE TWELVE STEPS FOR HEALTHCARE

Now that you know a little more about the principles of recovery, I'd like to take a moment to further discuss the Twelve Steps. Originally written as a path to healing from substance use disorders, these simple and profound principles have helped tens of millions of people worldwide rebuild their lives with honesty, humility, and community at the center.

Throughout this book, we've been applying the wisdom of recovery not just to individuals, but to the healthcare system itself. We've identified that the problem is more than just burnout, broken workflows, or strained relationships. It stems from a deeper disconnection from our collective values and from each other.

So, what if we took the Twelve Steps and reimagined them as a framework for recovering healthcare? They may not all resonate with you right away, but I encourage you to sit with them. Revisit them. Reflect on how they show up in your own story, your team, and your institution. Because if we can begin to live these principles, we can start to heal ourselves and the culture of medicine.

1. Honesty

We begin by telling the truth about our limits, burnout, and the ways the system has distanced us from the reasons we entered medicine in the first place.

2. The Present Moment

We practice returning to what is actually happening now: the patient in front of us, the body we inhabit, and the moment we are living, not the one we are rushing toward or replaying behind us.

3. Surrender

We release the illusion that we, as healthcare professionals, are always in control. We start to understand what we cannot change in our daily work, and we find the courage to change the things we can.

4. Safety

We acknowledge that healthcare is saturated with trauma (for patients and clinicians alike) and that unaddressed trauma shapes behavior, culture, and care. As such, we learn to develop a trauma-informed approach and psychological safety for our colleagues, patients, and ourselves.

5. Community & Service

We reject isolation and competition, choosing instead to heal in relationship. We support our colleagues and learners by being honest about the messy, human parts of practicing medicine while allowing ourselves to be supported in return.

6. Gratitude

We intentionally notice what is meaningful, human, and sacred in this work, using gratitude to reconnect with purpose.

7. Integrity

We realign our actions with our values, recognizing that moral injury occurs when the gap between who we are and how we practice widens.

8. Hope & Uncertainty

We learn to stay present when answers are unavailable, offering companionship rather than false certainty and trusting that hope can exist without guarantees.

9. Humility

We loosen our attachment to being indispensable, infallible, or admired, and remember that good medicine doesn't require self-erasure or heroism.

10. Authenticity & Curiosity

We replace defensiveness with openness, allowing ourselves and others to ask questions, admit uncertainty, and grow without shame.

11. Forgiveness

We practice repair of relationships and of self, understanding that accountability and compassion can coexist.

12. Resilience

We redefine resilience not as enduring harm, but as building lives, systems, and cultures that allow clinicians to remain whole.

COMMENCEMENT

I'd like to end this book with a commencement address I wrote for one of the graduating medical school classes I had the pleasure of teaching. I began writing it during my most recent stay in treatment, a time marked by both reckoning and clarity. The inspiration came from a suffocating culture of silence at my former institution.

Unfortunately, I wasn't able to give this speech at graduation, for I had already moved on to work at another hospital. I was, however, able to share it with the students I mentored. I wanted to make sure they understood that it's ok to ask for help, especially as they entered one of the most challenging periods of their lives: residency training. The message was simple: *you don't have to go through it alone.*

I chose to end the book this way because commencement is not an ending; it's a new beginning—an invitation to start again. So, as you read these final pages, know this: the book may be over, but the real work is just beginning. It's the work of healing and changing a broken system from the inside out. The work of recovering healthcare - together.

I believe it's possible. I can see it on the horizon.

All it takes is a willingness to show up with honesty, with purpose, and with heart — one day at a time.

Dear Medical School Graduates,

My name is Tony. I'm an OBGYN hospitalist in the Department of Obstetrics and Gynecology. But more than that, I'm a teacher, a musician, a brother, a dog dad, an athlete, a son, and a very human, very imperfect gay man living in New York City.

I began writing this commencement address while on medical leave last fall. Some of you may know why. I live with a chronic illness, one that is often misunderstood, stigmatized, and still rarely spoken about in our profession. It's lifelong. It's complex. It's deadly. And like many chronic conditions, it comes with relapses and uncertainty.

I have a substance use disorder.

I am an addict.

And I am also a doctor.

So now that you know a bit more about me, let me reintroduce myself in the way I've come to know myself best:

Hi, I'm Tony, and I'm a recovering addict and alcoholic.

But addiction and medicine aren't my whole story. They are just part of the fabric of who I am. And that's why, when I work with students, residents, nurses, midwives, and physician assistants, I rarely introduce myself as "Dr. Grandelis." I simply say: "I'm Tony." That's it.

Because what I've learned in the rooms of recovery (and in every corner of the labor floor) is that healing doesn't happen in hierarchy. It happens in community. In partnership. In friendship. We make it through the hardest things in life together. We learn from each other. We laugh and grieve with one another. And we become better clinicians, better humans, by standing shoulder to shoulder, not top to bottom.

I need you just as much as you've needed me. I've learned from you. I've processed heartbreaking cases with you. I've been reminded on a daily basis why I do this work, and why it matters.

A huge part of my own struggle with addiction stems from a deep-rooted sense of not belonging. I grew up gay in the Midwest, constantly trying to hide the parts of myself that felt too different. I learned early on that survival sometimes meant shapeshifting. It meant performing. It meant shrinking.

By the time I reached third-year clinical rotations, those feelings came roaring back. I often felt like I didn't belong on the wards. I felt like I wasn't smart enough, fast enough, useful enough. I felt dispensable. Invisible. I questioned everything. I thought about quitting more than once. And then, just when I needed it most, someone would show up (an attending, a resident, a nurse) who reminded me I mattered. In the recovery world, we call that our higher power showing up.

And I'm so grateful I stayed. Because now I get to do the job I love most: Teach. Work alongside all of you. Watch you grow into the phenomenal physicians you are becoming.

But what does it mean to be a phenomenal physician?

I'm not sure there's one perfect formula. But I encourage you to look back. Think of the educators, mentors, or colleagues who left a mark on you. What made them special? What made them safe? What made you trust them?

For me, it's the people I've met in recovery, physicians and patients alike, who've shown me the most extraordinary examples of humanity. They've taught me that the greatest clinical virtues are not found in the pages of textbooks. They're found in Kindness. Patience. Compassion. Forgiveness. And Radical Acceptance.

These aren't just values I bring to my patients. They're the values I've had to learn—slowly, painfully—to offer myself.

The boy who didn't fit in... the student who doubted everything... the man who got sick... the doctor who relapsed... he, too, deserves grace.

And so do you.

We all have our demons. And when they feel too heavy to carry alone, I hope you remember this: You are not expected to be resilient all the time. Sometimes, resilience just isn't possible. And in those moments, strength is asking for help.

It's saying, "I'm not okay."

It's hitting pause so you can come back whole.

The work will be here when you return.

To those of you I've worked with, and especially to the eight of you I've had the deep privilege of mentoring this past year, I want to say: I am proud of you. Beyond words. You're stepping into a chapter that will be equal parts exhilarating and exhausting. You'll experience joy and heartbreak, triumph and self-doubt. And through it all, I hope you never forget your worth.

You are already remarkable. And you don't need awards or publications to prove that.

Do you want to know what keeps me going? It's you.

Your kind words. Your curiosity. Your courage.

When I read a thoughtful student evaluation after a hard week, it reminds me that I matter. That I still belong. That I have something to give.

So as you go forward, I ask one thing of you:

Remember the medical student on your team.

Look them in the eye. Invite them into the room. Show them they belong. Be the person they remember in their darkest hour.

Because sometimes, that one person makes all the difference.

Congratulations.

You made it.

And the world is better – will be better – because of you.

Thank You.

AFTERWORD

What to Do If You Are Concerned About a Colleague—Or Yourself

If you're reading this and find yourself wondering whether you, or someone you work alongside, might be struggling with a substance use disorder, I want you to pause and remember: There is help. There is hope. And there is a way forward.

Substance use disorders are treatable. Many healthcare professionals recover fully and return to fulfilling, meaningful lives and careers. I'm one of them. But the road to recovery, particularly in medicine, is often shadowed by stigma, fear, and silence.

We have to break that silence.

If You're Concerned About a Colleague

You are not alone in your concern, and you are not responsible for fixing the problem. You are also not responsible for reporting your colleague to a medical board or licensing authority. In fact, doing so prematurely may cause unnecessary harm, including the loss of a career that could otherwise be saved with appropriate support.

Here's what you can do:

- Speak to a supervisor you trust. This could be a department chief, program director, or wellness lead. If your institution has a physician wellness or impairment committee, they can confidentially help assess the next steps.
- Refer or report to your state's healthcare professional monitoring program (also called Physician Health Programs). These programs are designed to provide confidential, specialized support for doctors, nurses, and other licensed professionals struggling with substance use or mental health concerns.
- Be honest with the person. Let them know you're worried. Say, "I care about you, and I'm worried. You don't have to do this alone. Can we speak with [supervisor] together? There's a path forward, and people who can help."
- Never react with anger, mockery, or condescension. Substance use disorder is a disease, not a character flaw. Harsh or shaming reactions only drive the problem deeper underground and make recovery less likely.

WHAT ARE HEALTHCARE PROFESSIONAL PROGRAMS?

Healthcare professional monitoring programs are in place in nearly every U.S. state. Their mission is to protect the public while also supporting recovery and career preservation for healthcare workers facing mental health or substance use challenges.

Here's what these programs typically offer:

- Confidential evaluation and referral to treatment, often by addiction medicine experts who understand healthcare culture. They may recommend at least a 30-day inpatient treatment program, so do not be surprised by this. And do not be afraid of these programs. They are wonderful and have changed countless lives — including my own.
- Monitoring and support contracts, which may include random drug testing, workplace reporting, peer support, and therapy.
- Advocacy with employers and licensing boards, helping ensure that as long as participants follow their agreed-upon recovery plan, their licenses are protected, and reports to the board are often unnecessary.
- Return-to-work planning, ensuring that reentry into clinical care is safe, supportive, and well-structured.

These programs are rigorous, and for good reason. They are built to protect patients while also ensuring that providers in recovery have the structure, accountability, and support they need to thrive.

And here's the truth: they work. Recovery rates for physicians in these programs are remarkably high.

Please, don't wait for things to get worse. You don't have to hit rock bottom. You don't have to lose your license. You don't have to live in fear or isolation any longer.

Reach out. Start with a trusted colleague. Contact your state's Physician Health Program directly. Join a recovery meeting specifically for healthcare professionals. Ask for help. Someone will answer.

Addiction is not the end of your career. Through recovery, it might be the beginning of something deeper, stronger, more whole.

Final Thoughts

We cannot heal healthcare without healing ourselves and each other. If someone around you is struggling, be the voice of compassion. If you are the one struggling, let someone be that voice for you. You are not your illness. You are not your mistakes. You are not alone.

Recovery is possible.

Connect with the Author

info@anthonygrandelismd.com

anthonygrandelismd

Anthony Grandelis

anthonygrandelismd.com